STATE CHANGE

STATE CHANGE

End Anxiety, Beat Burnout, and
Ignite a New Baseline of Energy and Flow

Dr. Robin Berzin
with Sarah Toland

SIMON ELEMENT

New York   London   Toronto   Sydney   New Delhi

SIMON
ELEMENT

An Imprint of Simon & Schuster, Inc.
1230 Avenue of the Americas
New York, NY 10020

First Simon Element hardcover edition January 2022

SIMON ELEMENT and colophon are trademarks of Simon & Schuster, Inc.

For information about special discounts for bulk purchases, please contact Simon & Schuster Special Sales at 1-866-506-1949 or business@simonandschuster.com.

The Simon & Schuster Speakers Bureau can bring authors to your live event. For more information or to book an event, contact the Simon & Schuster Speakers Bureau at 1-866-248-3049 or visit our website at www.simonspeakers.com.

Interior design by Jennifer Chung

Manufactured in the United States of America

1   3   5   7   9   10   8   6   4   2

Library of Congress Cataloging-in-Publication Data
Names: Berzin, Robin, author.
Title: State change : the new science of ending anxiety, beating burnout, and reaching a higher baseline of energy and flow / Dr. Robin Berzin.
Description: First Simon Element hardcover edition. | New York, NY : Simon Element, 2022. | Includes bibliographical references and index.
Identifiers: LCCN 2021026971 (print) | LCCN 2021026972 (ebook) | ISBN 9781982176808 (hardcover) | ISBN 9781982176822 (ebook)
Subjects: LCSH: Anxiety disorders—Treatment.
Classification: LCC RC531 .B44 2022 (print) | LCC RC531 (ebook) | DDC 616.85/22—dc23
LC record available at https://lccn.loc.gov/2021026971
LC ebook record available at https://lccn.loc.gov/2021026972

ISBN 978-1-9821-7680-8
ISBN 978-1-9821-7682-2 (ebook)

This book is dedicated to my patients,
and to all the patients at Parsley Health,
whose stories of healing are why I do what I do.

✳

CONTENTS

CHAPTER ONE   The True Secret to Transformation   1

CHAPTER TWO   How You Really Feel   21

CHAPTER THREE   What Your Life Is Doing to Your Brain   45

CHAPTER FOUR   The Diagnostic Tests You Really Need   65

CHAPTER FIVE   Move the Energy   95

CHAPTER SIX   Food for Energy, Focus, and Flow   117

CHAPTER SEVEN   The Universal Addiction Killing
                   Our Minds and Draining Our Mood   159

CHAPTER EIGHT   Supplements to Change Your
                   Energy and Flow   187

CHAPTER NINE   The New Frontiers: Psychedelics,
                   Meditation, and Energy Healing   211

CHAPTER TEN   Putting Words to Work: A Thirty-Day Plan
                   to Reset Your Mind and Mood   233

                   Acknowledgments   255

                   Bibliography   257

                   Index   285

CHAPTER ONE

The True Secret to Transformation

Two large coffees, skim milk, three Splendas, two dollars—it was the same every day. The guy behind the street cart outside my downtown New York City office knew my order without having to ask.

This was 2003. I had just turned twenty-one years old and was freshly out of college. In those days, I lived off this coffee concoction loaded with artificial sweetener, caffeine, and the hope it would somehow make my day go by faster.

As I sipped the coffee on a bench steps away from the subway entrance, the Financial District in downtown Manhattan in the month of September felt like a movie set to me: the smell of roasted nuts mixed with the taxi exhaust, people in suits no matter how sweltering the outside air, and the feeling that things were always beginning.

I should have felt like I had the whole world in front of me, but instead I was lost. Graduating summa cum laude and Phi Beta Kappa from an Ivy League university with a degree in international relations meant that I was really, really good at school—and not good at much else. I had learned to use my intellect as armor, always having the right answer, always making the right choice, justifying the wrong choices as right ones, and living perpetually in my head. Armed with this "I must have all the answers" outlook, I subsisted on a rinse-and-repeat combination of caffeine, red wine, and calorie restriction (in the body-dysmorphic way, not the biohacker way) that cycled me through days in the office and nights out partying. I was very far away from becoming the doctor, mom, and CEO I am today—in fact, I could never have imagined this kind of future then.

My first job out of college was as a paralegal in New York, where I prosecuted securities fraud for the US Attorney's Office. The job was a gift, and not just because it was a relatively distinguished opportunity for a recent college grad and came with the highest security clearance I will certainly ever have in my lifetime. It was a gift, because in a mere six months it showed me exactly what I didn't want to do with the rest of my life. While someone very smart should absolutely prosecute securities fraud on behalf of all Americans, I remember telling my best friend over drinks one night that I didn't think it should be me.

The "this is not working" feeling I had about my career was compounded by my romantic relationship at the time. I had been with the same boyfriend for almost three years, but we'd long cruised past the territory of "healthy relationship" into what I would describe as a wildly immature, dysfunctional, and competitive relationship. I regularly spent lunch breaks outside the office, tracing the paths of City Hall Park, sipping my fake-sugar-sweet street-cart coffee while crying and arguing with him on the phone.

In my early twenties, I survived on coffee, green apples from the farmers' market outside my apartment building, protein bars, and grilled chicken from the sandwich counter at my local bodega—no exaggeration. I unknowingly subscribed to the cult of orthorexia before the obsession with "healthy" eating became a thing. At the time, I had no pretenses around being "healthy." Instead, I just thought healthy equaled skinny.

To accomplish that end, I also ran on the treadmill at the YMCA three to four times a week, Z100 blasting in my headphones as I thought about which flavor of Tasti D-Lite I would reward myself with after my run. Being "healthy" to me simply meant fitting into a size Small while simultaneously subsisting on sugar in alcohol, protein bars, and fake sweeteners. I was doing well at work, and despite my crazy gone-on-too-long relationship with my boyfriend, I had a great social life, lots of friends, and endless evening plans. The lack of sleep, perma-hangover, daily brain fog, and mood swings didn't seem to me to be an issue. It's what we all did.

The only problem was that I didn't feel good. I was anxious, stressed, and lost, and without realizing it, I started to try to find a way out—of everything. On some visceral level I knew that I wasn't on the right path—I certainly wasn't on the path to become who I am today. But I had absolutely no idea where that path was or how to find it.

Like a mouse in a maze, I started walking, a lot. Initially, it was just around the neighborhood where I worked. My paralegal duties most days were manageable, so unless one of the cases I was responsible for was at trial, I had extra time on my hands, and walking took the place of sitting at my desk reading the *New York Times* online for the fifth time. A few months into my wanderings, I happened upon a flyer pasted to a streetlight on Warren Street. It was for $5 classes at a yoga studio in a fourth-floor walk-up above one of those jam-packed ground-floor shops in New York City that has a little of everything—staplers, screwdrivers, Halloween costumes. The neighborhood was slowly coming back to life after 9/11, and my first three classes were going to be only $15. This was attractive because I was broke (my government paralegal salary barely paid the rent), and I signed up because I needed something to do when I didn't feel like window shopping or crying on the phone. I knew nothing about yoga—the practice was hardly standard curriculum for college students in those days, and my upbringing in Baltimore had emphasized team sports like soccer and lacrosse instead.

I was skeptical of yoga at first. The studio was only one room, and you changed behind a curtain. The windows had been retrofitted with stained glass. Was this a church? The people in class, mostly women, were older than me for the most part and appeared to be very fit, but not in the skinny Splenda-wine-and-coffee way. They actually looked strong. I wasn't sure that I was supposed to be there, because it felt like they all knew one another. But I had nothing better to do.

Yoga was immediately different from running on the treadmill at the Y. My breathing slowed. My focus stayed in the room. I discovered that holding still was more difficult than moving quickly. After the thoughts stopped racing through my head, I became acutely aware of my body in space for the first time. My sweat felt like it was coming from a deeper place than just below the surface of my skin.

It wasn't just energizing—it was also frustrating. I realized that I had no core strength whatsoever. I learned that while I was great at moving forward through time and space, I was terrible at balancing in the here and now, as I fell over simply trying to stand on one foot for several seconds. The "Om"-ing was weird and awkward, and the corpse pose, which meant lying around on the ground doing nothing, felt like a waste of time for a workout class. I had no idea what the Sanskrit words meant, just that I felt a little too woo-woo for even being in a room where they were said out loud.

After my first class, I threw my drenched clothes in a bag. It wasn't hot yoga; the class had just been that hard. As I walked back down the four flights of stairs, I noticed a strange feeling. First, my legs were shaking like I'd just run ten miles. Second, I was calm, possibly for the first time ever. My head wasn't spinning through that cycle of external blame and internal shame that I'd been stuck in for years—the same one I had used to rationalize my reality. Instead, I felt suddenly in the present, without worrying about what was going to happen next or reexamining everything that had already happened in the hopes of reaching a different outcome. That feeling of constant tension, like my body was attached to a live wire, was gone. I felt free.

While I didn't appreciate it at the time, I had just used my body to change my mind—I had used my physiology to overhaul my psychology. This wasn't just a quick fix, feel-good moment: This was the beginning of a transformation of my baseline emotional state leveraged by a shift in my physical state.

This metamorphosis of your emotional and mental health triggered by a change in your physical health is what I call a *State Change*. A State Change is when you establish a new normal, or a new set point for how you feel on a daily basis. At baseline, you feel happier, have an easier time discovering what you want, are able to tap into your passions, feel more confident in your decisions, and are able to unlock a new level of consciousness that you may have never realized even existed.

State Changes don't happen after one yoga class. But for me, one yoga class was the unexpected first step toward rethinking my daily behaviors, or core actions, as I call them throughout this book: the things we do every day with or to our bodies that can have a huge impact on our physical and mental health.

After my first yoga class, I found myself going back for a second and a third. After ten classes or so—and a similar experience following each one—I became fascinated by the connection between my mind and my body. I hadn't ever known

I could feel so clear, present, calm, and connected. The feeling lasted far beyond the hour-long class, influencing the way I saw my life and myself. Yoga was still weird to me, and I routinely made fun of it to my friends, but I found myself going back again and again, searching for that feeling and the consequential confidence that seemed to magically result.

My first State Change led to a major shift that ultimately changed my life. This started, though, with a physical, mental, and emotional wake-up call. Suddenly, I realized just how many of my waking hours were spent in a continual state of distraction and anxiety, as I began to discover through yoga more clarity, energized calm, and mindfulness. Eventually, a calmer, more energized state wasn't just my in-class mode but my new baseline—how I felt on a consistent, regular basis. Unlike other types of exercise where I felt exhausted afterward or like I was literally and figuratively stuck on a treadmill, yoga showed me how to slow down, enjoy the moment, and feel more comfortable in my skin. The practice helped me see that my body wasn't the enemy—something I had to beat into shape or force to tone up or whittle down—but a beautiful vehicle for movement. I started to focus on feeling strong rather than making sure I worked out for a certain amount of time, lifted X pounds of weights, or burned Y number of calories.

But it wasn't just about yoga—or even exercise in general. After my first State Change, I began to examine other core actions—the foods I regularly ate, how I slept, how and how much I stared at screens—and ways I might be able to shift these core actions, like I had done with exercise, to achieve a State Change on another level. In particular, I started paying attention to how certain foods made me feel, as I realized many of the things I consumed on a regular basis left me feeling wired, tired, or bloated. Similar to exercise, I began to see that I had been using food for the wrong reasons—to be skinny, for example, not to feel more vibrant, alive, calm, and comfortable in my digestion. As I experimented with what I ate, I began to understand there were lots of ways to have a State Change. I didn't have to start or stick with exercise—I could use any core action to achieve a new baseline. These core actions, or what I did daily with my body, weren't just a "lifestyle," which had always seemed like a wishy-washy concept, but doorways I could open to feel better, healthier, and happier.

My State Changes weren't just physical, mental, and emotional. After I discovered a new baseline with yoga, I found myself reevaluating what I wanted to do with the rest of my life (surprise, federal prosecution was not my future), not from a place of fear but rather from a place of tapping into the things I now cared about. The first was a new interest in health. So in the summer of 2004, I quit my paralegal job and started working in the psychiatric research unit at NYU's School of Medicine.

I also stopped running like my life (and my weight) depended on it. I broke up with the boyfriend—eventually. And over the next year, I slowly cut out all the calorie-counting and fake sugars and began to eat real meals. Amazingly, I was shocked to find I still fit into my jeans. Actually, they fit even better, as I discovered I was far less fixated on the number inside the waistband.

I also discovered that I liked working in psychiatric research at the Manhattan Veterans Administration hospital. I liked administering EKGs and drawing blood. I liked interviewing patients. I liked learning about brain scans. It was work with a purpose that felt helpful, not punitive. I liked my colleagues, too. I didn't have time to wander or be lonely, although I did work it out with my boss to come in early—7 a.m. most days—so that I could leave by 4 p.m. to make it to 4:15 p.m. yoga in FiDi.

One day, as I was getting coffee at a bodega on Twenty-Third Street during my walk from the 6 train to work, I found myself in line behind a middle-aged woman ordering a large coffee with skim milk and two Splendas. "I don't mean to pry," I told her, "but that stuff will kill you." She looked at me evenly for a beat. I thought she was going to tell me to mind my own business. But before I could mumble "Sorry," she turned back to the counter and said, "Never mind about the Splenda." She then looked at me, smiled, and said, "Bless you."

This is when I began to turn the intellectualism I had once used as a shield into a key, plying it to get into medical school at Columbia. I worked hard to earn my medical degree and finish my residency before deciding I could do better than just medicate and operate: I wanted to help people get truly better. I wanted to find and treat the root causes of physical pain and emotional distress. I wanted to help patients discover how wonderful life could be—and feel—when they no longer had to rely on caffeine, alcohol, sugar, and/or addictive drugs. Most of all,

I wanted to help them experience their own physical-emotional transformations that I knew would change their lives like my own transformation had already changed mine. It would be years before I knew enough about medicine to actually help people make these changes through testing, medications, and science, but my "why" was set, and I was on my path.

Now it's your turn. I believe that a more impassioned, empowered, energetic, and healthier life is possible, no matter who you are or what you're dealing with. You can have a State Change. And it all starts with one thing: your body.

The Big Problem with the Health Issues We All Have

F41.9. R53.83.

They may look like model numbers for the next Android phone, but there's nothing cutting-edge about them. They're medical classification codes—F41.9 for an anxiety diagnosis, R53.83 for general fatigue.

I know them like my own phone number because they're the two most common diagnosis codes used at my medical clinic, despite the fact that most patients come see me for physical problems like migraine headaches, gastrointestinal conditions, arthritis, and hormone imbalances.

I don't hand out these codes like candy because I like to play part-time shrink. Quite the opposite: I care about how my patients feel, both physically *and* emotionally. I also screen for anxiety, depression, sleep disorders, and general fatigue as part of our general intake process.

That's not standard practice at most primary care offices, but Parsley Health, which is the medical clinic I started in 2016 that now sees tens of thousands of patients across the country, is not a standard practice. At Parsley, we want to know as much about your mood, ability to focus, and whether you can find joy, as we do about your blood pressure and bowel movements. If your doctor isn't also asking you these types of questions, I can't say I'm surprised—but you may want to find a new doctor.

Some patients want to know why I'm so interested in their mental and emotional health. I tell them that if you're anxious, depressed, not sleeping well, or tired all the time, getting rid of that stomach problem you came in for is going to be much more difficult, if not impossible.

More important, there's a good chance that your stomach problem—whether it's from an ulcer because you're not dealing with your stress, or an imbalance in gut bacteria because you're eating too much sugar—is what's causing you to feel anxious, depressed, restless, or tired all the time in the first place.

F41.9 and R53.84 aren't the only diagnoses that are populating our patient records like suggested passwords, either—there are also the codes for brain fog, burnout, depression, attention deficit hyperactivity disorder, and insomnia. And this isn't just happening at Parsley Health—it's a phenomenon that's happening everywhere.

Feeling like general crap is so pervasive, in fact, that in 2018, the World Health Organization added "burnout" as a diagnosable medical condition (Z73.0 for the code-curious). Today, more than 90 percent of US workers say they feel burned out, as if they can't wake up and don't have the will or a way to try.

The stats on other aspects of our mental and emotional health are similarly staggering. For example, one in five Americans has clinical anxiety. One in twelve has major depression. Ten percent of all kids are diagnosed with ADHD, a condition that doesn't magically disappear on someone's eighteenth birthday.

These numbers reflect only those who seek help and get a clinical diagnosis as a result. In reality, the prevalence of these mental health issues is much higher, because most people don't raise their hand and ask for help from anyone, let alone a doctor—and if they do, too often no one is there to help them, given the shortage in mental health services.

Outside of clinical diagnoses, one in every three Americans doesn't get enough sleep, which may be why three-quarters of us say we feel tired all the time at work. In 2018, 13 percent of the country also reported feeling unhappy—a more than 50 percent uptick since 1990.

Unfortunately, the coronavirus pandemic hasn't done anything to help our national emotional health emergency. Instead, the outbreak has practically put anxiety, depression, and stress into the public water supply. In spring 2020, some experts estimated that the crisis had produced depressive symptoms in at least half of all Americans.

Pandemic or not, there are more Americans suffering from at least one emotional issue than there are people in this country with almost any other medical condition. And the problem is, no one is calling out our anxiety and feelings of being burned out or bummed out as a public health crisis. On the contrary, we've normalized these conditions simply as consequences of modern American life. They're part of our collective low baseline.

For proof, look inside the goldfish bowl of pop culture. Which celebrity, CEO, or similarly high-profile person isn't anxious, depressed, or teetering on the edge of total burnout? Everyone from entertainers like Oprah Winfrey and Robin Williams to business tycoons like Sir Richard Branson and Charles Schwab to world leaders and members of the British royal family has admitted to suffering from various mental health problems, including depression, anxiety, and burnout. While it's amazing these issues aren't actually stigmatized for celebrities in mainstream media, what's not so great is that we've come to accept these conditions as hallmarks of what happens when you try too hard to get everything you want in life.

Imagine if a friend told you that she never once felt stressed, tired, burned out, sad, anxious, or unfocused. You would probably either accuse her of lying or wonder how she managed to quit her job, move to Bali, and forgo all her other responsibilities.

Not only is this perspective deeply troubling, it's also total BS: Feeling anxious, tired, burned out, sad, and unable to focus should not be the new normal—and it's certainly not what you need to sustain if you want to be a functioning member of the twenty-first century and balance your career, family, and personal life all at once.

Flipping the Script on the Mind-Body Connection

So, why are we all so anxious, tired, burned out, and depressed? And what can we do about it?

From my experience as a physician, the answer to the first question, paradoxically, isn't in our heads. The reason so many of us suffer from emotional health issues, whether we've been diagnosed or not, isn't because life is inherently more stressful today or because our jobs are that much more difficult. Quite the opposite: Technology and other modern-day advancements have in some ways made life easier now than ever before.

What has changed, however, is not what's happening *around* us but what's happening *inside* us. Compared to several decades ago, we now consume more sugar (an average of sixty pounds per year), are far less active (sitting up to ten hours per day, with only 23 percent of us getting enough exercise for general health), stare at screens for twelve hours, take an average of four prescription drugs, and are exposed to hundreds of toxic chemicals in our diet and environment every day. None of these factors existed to this degree even thirty years ago, and these fundamental changes are the real reason so many of us feel sad, sick, and tired, despite our best efforts not to be sad, sick, and tired.

In other words, the root of our emotional health issues is our physical health—or lack thereof.

I see this every day in my patients. High-sugar diets are the norm for most, even though subsisting off sugar, whether directly in sweets and soda or indirectly in refined carbs, creates blood-sugar imbalances and brain inflammation that can lead to anxiety and depression. Exercise may fight bad mood as effectively as antidepressants, but most of us aren't doing anything active, as we sit and look at screens all day. Our smartphones are also problematic because they're addictive, activating the same brain receptors as cocaine to create daily highs and lows, reinforce feelings of inadequacy, and even atrophy the brain's gray matter. Our air, water, food, and personal-care products are filled with pollutants, hormone disruptors, and heavy metals, all of which erode cognitive function. And sleep—forget about sleep. Between caffeine, alcohol, stimulants, screens, and light and noise pollution in our bedrooms, almost none of us sleep long enough or well enough, which leads to more brain fog, sugar addiction, anxiety, and depression even in those who are otherwise healthy. These are the current core actions that are causing many people's baseline, or set point, for how we feel on an everyday basis, to be so dismally low.

All this means that we are a set up for sickness, physically. All you need to do is take one look at the US's skyrocketing rates of chronic illness like diabetes and arthritis, which now collectively account for 90 percent of our annual $3.5 trillion healthcare costs. But no one is paying attention to how our physical state is changing our mental and emotional health.

This includes no one in modern medicine, in my experience.

You would think that, given all the advancements in healthcare these days, doctors should be able to treat whatever physical issues we have if those issues are, in fact, causing us to feel burned out, bummed out, and anxious at an alarming rate.

But in reality, conventional healthcare is the reason so few of us are able to sustainably remedy our emotional problems. I'm not saying your doctor is causing your depression, fatigue, burnout, ADHD, or anxiety. But all too often, he or she isn't helping you solve the root of the problem, either.

Here's why. In conventional medicine, mental health and physical health are siloed into two separate buckets. If you have a mental or emotional problem, you see a psychiatrist or a psychologist; if there's something wrong with you physically, you see a primary care doctor or a specialist.

While I was doing my medical training at Columbia University and Mount Sinai Hospital in New York City, for example, if someone came into our primary care clinic and was identified as having a mental or emotional health issue, we referred them out to the psych clinic, which usually involved a month or longer wait. If a patient was hospitalized for a heart attack but also had anxiety, we'd call a psych consult to make a recommendation—and if we determined that severe anxiety had precipitated the heart attack, this patient was moved to the psych floor and no longer considered our problem. From the very first days of my medical training, I was taught that emotional and behavioral issues were not my department. Literally: not my department.

It works the other way, too. Psychiatrists are trained medical doctors, with the capability to order medical tests, do physical exams, and treat the body as much as they do the mind. But very few, if any, do these things. Instead, they typically say "not my territory" and refer patients with physical problems to primary care doctors. We get these kinds of referrals all the time at Parsley, where we'll diagnose a thyroid imbalance as the true cause of a patient's depression, caffeine or alcohol abuse as the real cause of another's insomnia or chronic migraines, or sleep deprivation as the ultimate reason for someone's anxiety.

Of course, psychological trauma and genetics can each be big factors in mental health issues, too, and not all such issues can be solved at the physical level. But what never ceases to amaze me is that the psych community ignores the physical as being either a possible cause of the problem or, at minimum, a helpful part of the solution. Because, again, it's not their department.

In reality, there's no magic concrete wall separating our minds from our bodies. And in medicine, if we're not looking at the full picture, we aren't playing with a full deck of cards.

Our mind, cognitive function, and emotional state are all part of a complex physical ecosystem that functions and thrives as one: body and brain, mind and emotions, thoughts and actions. None can be neatly siloed or separated out.

Aha, the mind-body connection! you think. But this book isn't about that. The mind-body connection, which states that our mind influences our body, is 100 percent valid, but it's also 100 percent unidirectional.

What we need to do is flip the script. This book is about how mental and emotional health is rooted in physical health—a truth that's been ignored by both conventional medicine and the psych community. It's about the fact that as much as the mind informs the body, the body also informs the mind.

In other words, our physiology determines our psychology. And if we truly want to get to the bottom of why so many of us feel tired, anxious, burned out, and bummed out, we need to step back and take a comprehensive, holistic look at what's really going on inside our bodies.

I take this comprehensive, holistic look with each and every one of my patients. Because of this approach, I'm able to help them resolve or improve long-standing mental or emotional health issues, often without medication. In fact, data from Parsley shows that we reduce patient reliance on psychiatric drugs by 47 percent. This isn't to say that these medications—the Zolofts, Prozacs, Xanaxes, and Ambiens of the medical world—aren't powerful tools that have an important place in our practice. They do, and we prescribe them; they can be lifesaving. But let's be honest: No one is lying awake at night because they're suffering from an Ambien deficiency. By looking deeper and putting nutrition, sleep, movement, toxin exposure, and technology onto the prescription pad alongside meds, we've helped thousands of people improve—and even cure—their mental health issues.

Most of medicine doesn't take the comprehensive, holistic view we do at Parsley, though. Despite the fact that food and lifestyle are responsible for 90 percent of all medical outcomes, both are treated as immaterial by our medical system—or at least as someone else's department. When was the last time you picked up a prescription for more green vegetables and eight hours of sleep, taken daily for at least three months? Never. This is one reason so many of us lack clarity, focus, energy, and optimism, not to mention why 60 percent of us suffer from at least one chronic illness, like cancer (50 percent of which is preventable, according to the National Cancer Institute), diabetes, rheumatoid arthritis, or heart disease.

Rather than treating our daily core actions like what we eat, how we move, and how much we stare at screens, conventional medicine pulls the same two arrows from its favorite combined quiver: prescription drugs and invasive procedures. While drugs and procedures are absolutely necessary at times, when either is prescribed without investigating the root cause of a medical problem—mental, emotional, or physical—it's like slapping a Band-Aid on a bleeding wound without addressing what triggered the hemorrhage in the first place. That's not an especially effective strategy.

Today, the prescription drug industry is a $600 billion annual money grab. Approximately two-thirds of all Americans take at least one prescription drug, while more than half of the US population over age sixty-five takes at least four prescription medications. While this is great news for Big Pharma, it's terrible news for the rest of us, because these drugs aren't solving our problems in many instances but are just leaving us overmedicated and undertreated.

In other words, the healthier we try to be, the sicker we get. Unfortunately, this is how American healthcare works. I want to show you how to overcome conventional healthcare's limitations in order to transform your mental and emotional health without waiting for the system to catch up.

I'll give you an example. I had a patient at Parsley who was in her forties, living in New York City, and working a typical desk-jockey job. Nothing was particularly unusual about her life, but at the same time, everything was wrong with it. She came to see me because her doctor had prescribed her statins, blood thinners, and Zoloft to treat her high cholesterol, high blood pressure, and depression, respectively. But despite swallowing this fistful of pills every day for years, she wasn't getting any better. She was also overweight and couldn't seem to lose fat no matter what she did.

When I saw her at Parsley, I didn't just run some basic blood work or try to find another prescription drug that might work better. Instead, I took a holistic view and looked at everything from her emotional health to her nutritional habits and other daily core actions to assess whether she might have a nutritional deficiency or underlying medical condition. What I found was that she was subsisting on a high-sugar diet (common), had a thyroid problem no one had tested for (common), and was sitting all day in front of a screen without any daily movement, let alone dedicated exercise (common).

I suggested she make a few simple changes to her nutrition and started treating her thyroid issue, and our health coach taught her how to move more throughout the day while cutting back on her screen time, all without asking her to quit her job or become a full-time gym rat. Several months later, not only was she clinically healthier, she also felt better. Her cholesterol and blood pressure had normalized, and her depression had improved. She had also dropped twelve pounds without even one day of the diet-and-deprive mentality she had for years associated with weight loss.

This story shows us that if you want to end anxiety, fatigue, and burnout and finally feel *really* good—not just okay or able to get through the day or surviving but actually energized, optimistic, and focused—you have to understand that your body is a fundamental driver of your emotional health. Once you wake up to this fact, something truly powerful happens: You unlock a huge potential to change how you feel, right here and now, regardless of whether you have a doctor willing or even able to help you.

It doesn't matter if you have a clinical diagnosis for depression, burnout, ADHD, insomnia, or anxiety—most of us aren't formally diagnosed, but many of us still suffer from these conditions to some degree; they're part of being human. What matters is that you're willing to make small, simple changes to help yourself. So many people have fallen into the chasm of feeling crappy, emotionally and physically, and conventional medicine isn't going to pull them out. You might have to climb out on your own. And I'm going to help you.

Starting with Your Story

It was our first appointment together, and Alyssa, thirty-four, was sitting on my exam table, sobbing. I could see why. She had been dealing with severe bloating, gas, headaches, and brain fog for years. The migraine medication another doctor had prescribed for her headaches was making her dizzy, and the ADHD drug Adderall, which she took for brain fog, had only made her digestive issues worse. Pulling at a tear-and-snot-soaked tissue in her hand, Alyssa said she was worried these drugs would interfere with her ability to have a baby and that she didn't feel old enough to be struggling with such persistent health problems.

As she talked through her tears, I knew what was wrong with Alyssa before I even examined her. As part of Parsley's intake process, all new patients like Alyssa complete an online health biography before they show up for their first visit. Our health biography isn't like any other doctor's form you've ever filled out. I essentially want all my new patients to tell me their entire life story. Because your entire life story is also the story of your health.

As part of your health biography, I want to know every influential event that's happened to you physically, medically, and emotionally since the day you were born. I want to know whether you were born vaginally or by C-section, the foods you ate growing up, the illnesses you had at ages five, fifteen, thirty-five, fifty-five—whenever—the medications you've taken from the time you were an infant until today, and even how willing you are to make changes to your personal life. In other words, I want the entire story of you, because that story is what created the person who walks into my doctor's office with troubling symptoms and/or general malaise.

Back to Alyssa: After reviewing her health biography, I knew she had taken antibiotics for sinus infections for most of her twenties. Her diet was also mostly made up of sugar and low-quality carbs, even though she assumed she was eating "healthy" because she was consuming things like low-calorie yogurt and gluten-free bread—the mid-2010s version of protein bars, aka high-sugar convenience foods green-washed as "healthy." She didn't connect her digestive issues to her headaches or brain fog, and no one had ever tied what was going on in her body and mind today with what had happened in her body and mind in the past.

But Alyssa's symptoms didn't just fall out of the sky and suddenly hit her over the head last week. While the antibiotics she had taken throughout her twenties might have killed off the bad bacteria causing her sinus infections, I knew they had also devastated her body's population of good microbes that she needed for healthy digestion. A long-standing microbiome imbalance was why she felt bloated and gassy today and was also contributing to her constant headaches and brain fog. I could have doubled her dose of Adderall and migraine medication, but I knew it wouldn't stop her symptoms because it wouldn't address the root cause of her problems: her gut.

At the end of our appointment, I sent Alyssa to get a specialized breath test to see what was going on inside her GI tract. Even though it was early in our process, I didn't necessarily need to see the test results to know what was going on. I knew that Alyssa likely had small intestine bacterial overgrowth (SIBO), caused by years of antibiotic overuse, and that she was addicted to sugar—a dietary drug she used to try to relieve her headaches and brain fog, but which had only perpetuated her microbiome imbalance.

Alyssa's health issues weren't the bad-luck hand she believed her body had dealt her at age thirty: They were the result of her life story, and conditions that had been written into her body years ago. By telling me her story, Alyssa was able to get off the medications, clean up her diet, restore her gut health, and finally end her indigestion, brain fog, and headaches. Today, she's focused, clear-headed, and symptom-free—and the mother of a healthy baby boy.

Alyssa's story illustrates what I tell all my patients: No matter what happened in the past, how long you've been sick, or how sick you are, ownership of your health starts now. *Now* could be when you're eighteen years old or when you're sixty years old. You may have grown up in a food desert, without access to healthcare, or with a genetic predisposition to heart disease. You could have a diagnosis of cancer or Lyme disease, have been in a car accident that required surgery, or have a history of psychological trauma leading to depression. None of these conditions or diagnoses are your fault or could have been prevented, and there's no shame or blame in them. But while they may not have been under your control and there's nothing you could have done to prevent them at the time, there's almost always something you can do differently now to change the trajectory of your future.

Taking ownership of unfortunate things without feeling shame is missing in our culture—which, to me, is the biggest shame. Taking responsibility of your health right now—good or bad—and acknowledging what you know about the state of your body and mind are empowering actions. As far as I'm concerned, you can leave shame at the door, as it's not a helpful sidekick for this journey. Once you know what you need to do to improve your health, you know. And from there, you have the opportunity every day to rewrite the story of your physical, mental, and emotional health with the foods you eat, the medicines you take, the exercise you do (or don't do), the kind of sleep you get, the way you deal with stress, and the other core actions and behaviors you incorporate into your being through your time and your dollars. No matter what you've done with your life up until this moment, the core actions and behaviors you choose from this day forward can reshape your future narrative, influencing your physical, mental, and emotional health for years to come.

I've always been clear about the fact that the story of your health is the story of your life. Ninety-nine percent of our health happens to us outside a doctor's office, while we're eating, sleeping, moving, going to work, interacting with other people, swallowing prescription drugs or supplements, and getting exposed to toxins in our air, water, food supply, and general environment. If you're my patient and I'm going to understand your health, I need to know what is happening and has happened to you outside my exam room—today and every day since you were young.

In functional medicine, a paradigm that informs the way I practice, doctors use an acronym called ATMs (antecedents, triggers, and mediators) to help determine the root cause of a patient's symptoms. I like ATMs because it's another way of getting people to think about their life story.

Here's how it works:

Antecedents are the conditions that predate your symptoms. Sometimes they can be genetic, but many times they are core actions, like what you eat, your exercise habits, technology consumption, and prescription-drug use. They might also include a specific event that laid the groundwork for you to start feeling unwell—for example, if you made a hectic move to a big city in your twenties or had a major surgery in your thirties, either incident could have driven up your stress levels and driven down your sleep.

Triggers are what provoke symptoms. They include things like illnesses and infections, a bacterial imbalance, a major life event, or, as in Alyssa's case, a bout of prescription medications.

Mediators are the daily core actions that sustain your symptoms, making it impossible for you to get rid of them. For example, if you're continuing to eat the same foods that helped derail your intestinal health years ago or are staring at screens for ten hours a day and wondering why you might still have headaches, these are the mediators that are likely keeping the lid locked on your ability to overcome your issues.

I want you to start thinking about your own life story right now using the health biography below as a starting place. This is the way that you can begin to understand the story behind why you might feel the way you do now—mentally, emotionally, and physically. Telling your story, whether you share the information with a doctor or not, can help you uncover what may be wrong not only with your health but also in your life, and empower you to make the small but powerful changes that can finally help you feel focused, clearheaded, and happy.

In the following exercise, use your own words to answer the questions as honestly and thoroughly as you can. The story of you is not short, so take your time and think about each answer carefully for as long as you need to. If something pops into your head, even if it seems trivial, write it down: Everything can be important, even those details you might assume are not. Your health biography can be only for you if you choose so; the goal is simply to get your story out of your head and your heart and into a place where you can look at it, objectively and analytically, for clues that can ultimately help you understand where your health came from, where it is today, and how you can turn it into a new story tomorrow.

1. How do you feel now? Be as specific as possible, including any mental or emotional issues you may have, like brain fog, fatigue, anxiety, or general sadness.

2. When did you last feel well? Not just okay—I mean consistently great.

3. How long have you had the symptoms you feel today? Has it been weeks, months, or years? Can you pinpoint the time when your symptoms started? Have you had these issues your whole life? If not, when did they start?

4. What was happening in your life when you first began to feel unwell? For example, did you start a new job or begin traveling more frequently? Did you get sick, have surgery, or end up in the hospital? Did someone close to you enter or leave your life? Did you change your diet, exercise, or sleep for any reason?

5. What symptoms did you have when you first began to feel unwell? Be as specific as possible, including any ailments like digestive issues, headaches, body pain, anxiety, and insomnia. Among these symptoms, can you identify which manifested first, second, and so on?

Awesome. Now keep your answers someplace safe, because I'll be talking about your health biography throughout this book. Remember, it's an important story—perhaps the most important story that you can and will ever tell for your overall longevity and joy.

Before you tuck your answers away somewhere safe, take a good look at what you wrote and see if you can connect the dots, like you started to feel X symptom after you switched jobs or Y symptom shortly after starting a new medication. You may be able to identify patterns—like that your digestive problems correspond with low emotional periods in your life—but if you can't, that's okay. By the end of this book, you'll get there. The goal right now is to simply have your story down on paper. Because if you don't know what's happened in your life and with your health, no doctor or other medical professional will be able to know.

Now that we've looked at your past, it's time to take you inside the present and get to the bottom of how you really feel, right now.

CHAPTER TWO

How You Really Feel

Pooping your pants is for babies, not for grown men and women.

It may be easy to think that until it happens to you. While it's an indignity no adult should have to face, many do, including the petite, successful graphic designer sitting in my office several years ago.

Melanie was in her early forties and had been dealing with chronic gas, bloating, and diarrhea for longer than she could remember when she made her first appointment with me two years ago. She was a long-distance runner and jogged every day, but her sudden bouts of explosive diarrhea had become so unpredictable that she had switched to the treadmill to be near a bathroom when she worked out. She had seen doctors for the issue, of course, including three different gastroenterologists, who told her she had irritable bowel syndrome (IBS) without giving her any guidance for what to do about it. That's why she came to see me.

What she didn't come see me for, though, was her anxiety. Melanie had a psychiatrist to help her with that, she told me, one whom she'd been seeing for more than five years. Like nearly all of my new patients, she didn't see anything wrong with this arrangement. She assumed what was happening with her body had nothing to do with what was going on inside her mind. She also believed, like most new patients, that mental health issues took years to solve and that seeing the same therapist for five years without much improvement was normal. At the same time, Melanie thought doctors like me treated just the physical, and that her anxiety wasn't or shouldn't be my concern.

But the problem with this arrangement was that very little about Melanie's mind or body was actually getting addressed, never mind resolved. Despite the fact that she'd been on the antidepressant Zoloft for years, her anxiety hadn't improved significantly. She was still suffering from mild depression and had lost track of which foods made her feel bloated or worsened her diarrhea. Her relationship with food had hit at an all-time low.

Looking at Melanie across my desk, I saw a woman who was tired. Tired of feeling sick. Tired of being at war with her body. Tired of being tired. Her energy was like that of a war hero: skeptical, battle-weary, and difficult to impress, but at the same time, she was willing to still try whatever I could throw at her. She was here because she was ready for a change. This type of patient is often my favorite, but they can also be the most challenging: I knew that to help Melanie make any progress, I had to sit back, look at the whole picture, and begin connecting the dots.

Because the story of our health is the story of our lives, I knew that Melanie's aggregate symptoms were plot developments that had most likely been written years ago. I also had to understand more about her health than simply her bowel habits: I needed to know the way she lived, the illnesses she'd had, the medications she took (even when she was a kid), the foods she ate, and the other core actions she took or decisions she made with her body every day. I had to take a deep dive into her health biography.

What I discovered was that Melanie had been diagnosed with IBS back in high school. The common intestinal disorder, marked by gas, bloating, diarrhea, and intermittent constipation, seemed to launch a cascade of problems: After her IBS appeared, she developed depression. Her digestive issues made her self-conscious and uncomfortable in her body, which helped fuel her mood problems. As I walked her through her own story, I could see Melanie's eyes widen. She had never thought these areas of her life could be related, but I could tell that she was picking up what I was putting down.

As we talked, I learned that Melanie had been prescribed lithium in her twenties to help treat what psychiatrists believed to be a mood disorder. But the medication had left her with a low-functioning thyroid condition that had messed up her digestion even more. In her thirties, she had cycled on and off antibiotics for a couple of years to help treat recurrent urinary tract infections. Flash forward ten more years, and the community of bacteria inside Melanie's gut responsible for helping regulate digestion, otherwise known as the microbiome, was a mess.

As we wrapped up our first appointment, I explained that, even though we'd just spent an hour together going over her history, I still needed more data. I told her that the test results she had diligently brought from her last trip to a primary care doctor were useless to me. Melanie shot me side-eyes of skepticism, but her "tired of being sick and tired" feeling won out. She agreed to my asks: Get new blood work to assess her thyroid health, inflammation levels, and any possible nutrient deficiencies; have a breath test done to look for any overgrowth of bacteria in her upper gut; and undergo the infamous three-day poop test to evaluate her lower intestinal function. Not the most fun, but hey, it was worth it if she could avoid another pair of undies in the trash at the gym and yet another $3,000 colonoscopy that came back with no answers. And it was definitely worth it to run outside again.

When the results of all her tests came back, I wasn't surprised to learn that Melanie had an overgrowth of bad bacteria in her gut, likely caused by antibiotic overuse from all her UTIs. And it wasn't just bad bacteria: She also had an overgrowth of yeast in her intestines, thanks to the high-carb, high-sugar diet she was using to fuel her distance running.

The first treatment I recommended was that Melanie follow a gut-healing protocol that includes eliminating possibly inflammatory foods and taking targeted supplements for a little while. This protocol is basic 101 therapy for me and other providers at my practice, but it was nothing like anything she had ever tried before. The first step on the protocol is to remove all sugar and refined carbs from your diet, then eliminate gluten, other grains, and dairy, and, for at least a little while, cut out all alcohol. In addition to this diet, I started her on a regimen of medical-grade herbal supplements to help kill off the bad bacteria inside her gut, while also prescribing a prescription antifungal to counter the yeast overgrowth. At the same time, we addressed her thyroid problems by updating her medication regimen in that area.

Melanie and I set a date for a follow-up video call in six weeks. When I saw her on screen then, I was curious to know how she was doing on the new protocol. I knew she had seen her health coach since our last visit (at Parsley, health coaches are trained practitioners who work in tandem with doctors to help patients take the daily actions they need to overhaul how they feel). But the real work wasn't mine or the coach's—it was Melanie's. It's a big deal to fundamentally change your nutrition, let alone take supplements every day: You have to want to get better, and even then, it's a lot. But she had done it.

She was smiling on my screen for our video call. Her demeanor had notably changed. The jaded war hero had morphed into a triumphant silver-medal winner—literally, as she told me about winning second place in a half-marathon she had just completed. The digestion problems Melanie had had since high school—the same ones that had caused her so many embarrassing moments while running in Central Park and elsewhere in the city—were suddenly gone. She had totally reset her gut.

Something else was different about Melanie, too. As I asked my usual head-to-toe questions about how she was doing and oohed and ahhed over her transformed digestion, I realized that she was . . . happier. She told me she had begun to feel more comfortable and confident in her own skin. Without round-the-clock bloating, gas, and diarrhea, she no longer felt at war with her body, which allowed her finally to let go of her continual control over food. Since our mental health depends in part on the health of our microbiome, the dramatic shifts we had made in Melanie's gut using food, herbs, and medications had likely greatly improved her bacteria balance, influencing the chemicals her gut sent to her brain every day. She had bumped up her baseline to a new level, and her new everyday norm was happier, healthier, more confident, and more enjoyable.

Two months later, at our next visit, Melanie shared that she had successfully started to reintroduce gluten-free grains back into her diet, while her anxiety and depression continued to recede. In fact, she said, she wanted to try to reduce her daily dose of Zoloft. I don't take this kind of suggestion of a medication change lightly: She had been on the drug for a long time, and lowering her dose would have to be done gradually and carefully in order to avoid a setback. But I agreed to try, and over the next four months, we reduced her dose bit by bit, in the end lowering it to a quarter of her original prescription.

Not everything since has been sunshine and roses for Melanie, of course—she suffered a stressful incident at work last year that triggered a relapse of her anxiety—but the inevitable bad stuff that happens to us all doesn't affect her as much as it did in the past. Her everyday baseline is still much higher than before we started working together, and she knows she's in the driver seat of her body, mind, emotions, and, ultimately, her life.

The real reason Melanie was able to overcome so many of her symptoms—the mental ones as well as the physical—is because she finally broke down the metaphorical wall separating her body and brain to take a hard look at what could be causing all her problems and how they might be interrelated. While no doctor had connected her digestion and her anxiety, when I saw her I suspected the two were inseparable: In my experience, you can't heal one without addressing the other.

I want to make something clear: That Melanie hadn't ever connected her physical and mental health before wasn't her fault. How conventional medicine operates makes it easy for us all to insist on having this wall between our bodies and our brains. Medical doctors aren't trained to take care of the mental, emotional, or spiritual, while psychologists and psychiatrists aren't trained to investigate or even assess whether a mental problem may have a physical root.

There's another reason you're not to blame for being unable to get to the root cause of any symptoms you may be suffering, whether they're mental or physical: If you're like most people under age fifty, you probably don't have a primary care doctor, meaning you probably haven't seen a regular physician since your childhood pediatrician. This also means you likely haven't had regular blood work or other tests done to show whether your hormones are imbalanced, your blood sugar is dangerously close to prediabetic, or you have Crohn's disease—all common ailments among Gen Xers and millennials, despite our love of yoga, health apps, and kale. And even having a primary care doctor is no guarantee that any of these underlying health issues will be discovered, let alone resolved, since most doctors are trained to treat symptoms, not what's causing them.

If you're one of the few who actually has a primary care doctor, he or she probably outsources you to a specialist for issues beyond a basic cough, cold, or infection. Oftentimes, specialists take an even more myopic approach, focusing only on the one body part or physiological system in which that provider is trained. The way our healthcare system silos out symptoms, you've likely talked about your mental and emotional health only with a psychologist or psychiatrist, if you were lucky enough to get to one, and they probably didn't ask you anything about your physical health. This was certainly the case with Melanie, and with nearly all my other patients.

This isn't laziness on the part of your doctor—it's simply the way conventional medicine works right now. Over and over again, I see new patients come to me because they've hit a dead-end wall with their medical care: Nothing is getting better, not their physical symptoms and not their mental or emotional health. They tell me they feel stuck in a rut and continually stressed out, bummed out, or burned out.

And it's not for lack of trying on their end: Many new patients tell me they've been regularly seeing the same therapist for two, five, or even ten years. This is when I'll ask, without any judgment, whether they feel their mental health has improved in that time. Are their emotions simply being managed or is how they view the world actually changing, with the picture becoming brighter and more resilient? This is when many of my patients get this saucer-eyed look as they begin to realize that they don't feel any better or haven't made progress to where they want to be, despite the fact that many of them have been on medication or in therapy for years. Their lack of progress isn't a sign that their psychologist or psychiatrist is incompetent, but many times, no amount of therapy, even if it's super-insightful, can fix a mental or emotional issue with a physical root or that's somehow tied to what's going on inside your body.

How I help these patients who are stuck in a rut is what I want to do for you now. I want to help you get unstuck and realize a new baseline and level of mental (and physical) health that you may have not thought possible. I want to help you discover how your body is affecting your mind and give you the tools to discover how your physical and mental health are intricately en-twined. The first step to biohacking your overall health is to break down the wall that separates your body from your brain and take a hard look at how you really feel.

How Do You *Really* Feel?

Most of us don't know how we really feel—like *really* feel, inside our bodies and in our day-to-day mental and emotional health. Many of us have been so disconnected or cut off from what's happening inside our bodies and minds for so many years that we've lost our ability to recognize what's normal and what's not. We ignore commonplace symptoms like fatigue, headaches, indigestion, and weight gain until the wheels come off the wagon and we end up with a chronic illness or an outright medical emergency.

This is what happens time after time with patients who either ignore symptoms or suppress them with quick-fix, over-the-counter medications or prescription drugs. If we have a headache, for example, what is the first thing we often do? We pop an Advil. Constipated? Take laxatives. Acid reflux? Swallow a fistful of antacids. Bloating? We have Midol, diuretics, gas pills, or any combination of the three. The list goes on . . .

But the body's symptoms aren't pesky little distractions to be ignored, suppressed, or dealt with via whatever product we find at the pharmacy that promises instant relief. Symptoms might be annoying, but they're also critical pieces of information that you should take the time to listen to. They're your body's only way of waving the metaphorical red flag to say, *Hey, friend, pay attention. Something's wrong here.* They're our first warning signs of underlying issues like a hormonal imbalance, an unhealthy microbiome, an autoimmune disease, or a more serious condition that could be paving the way for a chronic illness like arthritis, diabetes, or even cancer.

While conventional medicine often waits until someone is riddled with symptoms or really sick in order to pronounce them sick, that's not why *you* picked up this book: You have the right, the opportunity, and the ability to prevent chronic disease, treat underlying issues, and live your life without fatigue, indigestion, pain, or any one of the other symptoms people often perceive as the inevitable side effects of modern life. In other words, you have the ability to have a State Change and move your everyday baseline out of the basement and onto the top floor.

To assess whether you might have an underlying issue or how your body is affecting your mind, though, you have to understand your body first—which means breaking down that wall and taking a hard look at how you really feel.

When I started Parsley Health, my team and I created something called the Parsley Symptom Index™, a full-body assessment that our team and I developed using FDA guidelines. (The PSI is a Patient Reported Outcomes Measurement developed and copyrighted by Parsley Health and cannot be copied, reprinted, changed, or modified.) It's the first and only medical questionnaire that helps people and their doctors connect the dots between a patient's symptoms and his or her overall health and well-being. The index allows patients to evaluate their symptoms holistically, as both individual signs and aggregate issues, to understand how different aspects of their health are interwoven and connected.

For many patients, using the PSI is an eye-opening experience. After they complete the questions, which take just a few minutes to finish, they realize they've been living with digestive issues, joint pain, skin problems, or other issues that they've either ignored or not recognized as having a big impact on their everyday well-being. Many discover their symptoms are part of a bigger problem they never knew they had, which might be the real reason they feel depressed, anxious, muddled, or mentally exhausted.

If you've completed a symptom questionnaire in the past and haven't had this kind of bombshell experience, I'm not surprised. Regular symptom trackers, like those given out at some doctors' clinics, aren't systematic or even in-depth, instead assessing if you're sick based on parameters like whether you can easily get out of bed in the morning. And if that's the gold standard of good health, I think we're all screwed.

The PSI is so unique that we've published it in peer-reviewed journals and used it to help tens of thousands of patients across the country figure out how they *really* feel. Short of coming to see me as a patient, using the symptom index is the best way to start to peel back what might be wrong and get to the bottom of how to use your body to change your mind and experience your first State Change.

The Tool to Help You Find Out How You Really Feel

Completing the symptom index beginning on page 32 asks you to assess your health over the past two weeks. It takes only two or three minutes, but when you complete it, you have the chance to connect with your body—a rarity for most people—and find out how you really feel.

Filling out the index will provide you with the baseline of how you feel right now. Then, when you repeat the index over time, you can see whether and in which ways your baseline changes, allowing you to identify potential hot spots, recognize connections between body systems, and track your overall health, with or without the help of a doctor. I recommend completing the index now and again in two to three weeks, and every month thereafter for six months' time.

When you repeat the PSI with regularity over time, you rule out one-off health issues that can throw off your score—for example, if you had a cold, did a hard workout, had a really stressful week, or ate some bad shellfish in the past two weeks, you may have symptoms you wouldn't normally experience. But if the same symptoms show up again and again, the issue probably isn't an isolated incident but information your body is trying to communicate to you. This is where the index provides a consistent, measurable way to connect with and listen to your body over time. And listening to your body is the first step to transforming how you feel, physically, mentally, and emotionally, and setting you up for a State Change.

Repeating the PSI over time also gives you a power typically reserved only for doctors: the ability to discover and recognize real patterns in your own health. Using the index, you can figure out if you're suffering from low-grade symptoms that you might not have realized you've had for a while—subtle or insidious things like fatigue, bloating, brain fog, and the other issues that so many of us have without recognizing our health is less than optimal. Why are we so unaware of the symptoms we have? It's difficult for almost any of us to remember how we felt two weeks or two months ago unless we take the time to ask ourselves how we feel and actually track our answers over time. I'm just as guilty: Half the time I can't remember what I ate for lunch yesterday, let alone if I had a headache or acid reflux last month. That's why I use the symptom index, too.

The index can also show you some pretty eye-opening patterns, like whether certain symptoms travel together, meaning they show up side by side. By completing the index more than once, for example, you may realize that you always feel bloated, get headaches, and have trouble sleeping at the same time, or are more likely to gain weight when your aches and pains flare up, which could indicate that your weight gain is tied to inflammation.

But it's not just that physical symptoms can go hand in hand with other physical symptoms: Mental and emotional issues can also manifest with certain physical symptoms—for example, you always feel depressed when you're constipated. This is where the symptom index is a huge value-add, since most people, including most doctors, can't or don't correlate mental symptoms with physical health. Again, it's not our fault: We've simply been conditioned not to connect what's going in our bodies with what's happening in our minds.

The index doesn't just track the bad—it can also help you evaluate what's going right, too. If you use the index over time in correlation with this book and begin to biohack your health with the tools outlined here, you can see which changes work best for you. This is an amazing advantage. Because so many of us can't remember how we felt last week or month, we often don't notice when we *stop* feeling tired, achy, or bloated. I see this all the time in my patients. They'll fill out the symptom index several months after their first appointment and are surprised to see that certain areas of their bodies don't light up like a lightbulb with symptoms anymore. I remind them how they felt when they first came to see me, and they're blown away. The index helps them see that what they're doing is working.

One thing to note: Completing the symptom index isn't meant to take the place of going to the doctor. If you have health concerns or symptoms that aren't improving, fill out the index, but also make an appointment with your healthcare provider. You can use anything you might discover by doing the index to help you and your doctor reach the right diagnosis.

The index also isn't meant to take the place of diagnostic testing, which is a critical component to unlock how your body might be affecting your mind (see Chapter Four on which diagnostic tests you may need and why). Testing is important, even if you feel fine, because many conditions don't manifest with symptoms until you're already seriously sick. For example, high blood pressure is called a "silent killer" because people usually don't feel anything until they suffer something traumatic, like a heart attack or a stroke.

What to Know Before You Complete the Symptom Index

The PSI assesses nine different body systems, or interrelated physiological areas, including reproductive health, which is specific to your biological sex. The nine body systems are represented by the index's nine numbered questions, and each body system includes five possible symptoms.

To complete the index, answer whether you've experienced any of the following symptoms in the past two weeks and, if so, the severity of the symptom, with 1 being extremely mild and 10 being the most severe you can imagine experiencing.

HOW TO RATE YOUR SYMPTOMS

- Symptom presence
    Yes: You're currently experiencing the symptom or have experienced it in the last 14 days
    No: You haven't experienced the symptom in the last 14 days
- Symptom severity (if symptom is present)
    1 - minimal
    2 - mild
    3 - uncomfortable
    4 - moderate
    5 - distracting
    6 - distressing
    7 - intense
    8 - unmanageable
    9 - severe
    10 - worst you can imagine

PARSLEY SYMPTOM INDEX (PSI)

1. In the last 14 days, have you experienced any of the following cardiac and circulatory symptoms:

* **Chest Pain**

Yes   No

1   2   3   4   5   6   7   8   9   1 0

* **Rapid or pounding heartbeat**

Yes   No

1   2   3   4   5   6   7   8   9   1 0

* **Lightheadedness or fainting**

Yes   No

1   2   3   4   5   6   7   8   9   1 0

* **Leg swelling**

Yes   No

1   2   3   4   5   6   7   8   9   1 0

* **Shortness of breath at rest**

Yes   No

1   2   3   4   5   6   7   8   9   1 0

Section subtotal: _____

2. In the last 14 days, have you experienced any of the following gastrointestinal symptoms:

* **Nausea or vomiting**

Yes   No

1   2   3   4   5   6   7   8   9   1 0

* **Heartburn or reflux**

Yes   No

1   2   3   4   5   6   7   8   9   1 0

* **Diarrhea or constipation**

Yes   No

1   2   3   4   5   6   7   8   9   1 0

* **Bloating or abdominal pain**

Yes   No

1   2   3   4   5   6   7   8   9   1 0

* **Excessive gas, flatulence**

Yes   No

1   2   3   4   5   6   7   8   9   1 0

Section subtotal: _____

3. In the last 14 days, have you experienced any of the following metabolic symptoms:

* **Abnormal weight gain or loss**

Yes   No

1   2   3   4   5   6   7   8   9   1 0

* **Intolerance to heat or cold**

Yes   No

1   2   3   4   5   6   7   8   9   1 0

* **Frequent urination**

Yes   No

1   2 .   3   4   5   6   7   8   9   1 0

✳ **Vision changes**

Yes   No

1   2   3   4   5   6   7   8   9   1 0

✳ **Excessive hunger or thirst**

Yes   No

1   2   3   4   5   6   7   8   9   1 0

Section subtotal: _____

4. In the last 14 days, have you experienced any of the following hair or skin symptoms:

✳ **Pimples or blackheads**

Yes   No

1   2   3   4   5   6   7   8   9   1 0

✳ **Abnormal hair changes**

Yes   No

1   2   3   4   5   6   7   8   9   1 0

✳ **Rashes (e.g., psoriasis, eczema)**

Yes   No

1   2   3   4   5   6   7   8   9   1 0

✳ **Abnormal nail changes**

Yes   No

1   2   3   4   5   6   7   8   9   1 0

✳ **Hives**

Yes   No

1   2   3   4   5   6   7   8   9   1 0

Section subtotal: _____

5. In the last 14 days, have you experienced any of the following neurological symptoms:

* **Headaches or migraines**

Yes   No

1   2   3   4   5   6   7   8   9   1 0

* **Fatigue or low energy**

Yes   No

1   2   3   4   5   6   7   8   9   1 0

* **Numbness, tingling, or other abnormal sensations (e.g., in hearing, taste)**

Yes   No

1   2   3   4   5   6   7   8   9   1 0

* **Sleep disturbances, difficulty staying asleep**

Yes   No

1   2   3   4   5   6   7   8   9   1 0

* **Memory changes (e.g., forgetfulness)**

Yes   No

1   2   3   4   5   6   7   8   9   1 0

Section subtotal: _____

6. In the last 14 days, have you experienced any of the following breathing/respiratory symptoms:

* **Wheezing, feelings of chest tightness**

Yes   No

1   2   3   4   5   6   7   8   9   1 0

* **Coughing**

Yes   No

1   2   3   4   5   6   7   8   9   1 0

✳ **Excessive mucus or nasal (sinus) stuffiness**

Yes   No

1   2   3   4   5   6   7   8   9   1 0

✳ **Snoring**

Yes   No

1   2   3   4   5   6   7   8   9   1 0

✳ **Irritated or sore throat**

Yes   No

1   2   3   4   5   6   7   8   9   1 0

Section subtotal: _____

7. In the last 14 days, have you experienced any of the following musculoskeletal symptoms:

✳ **Back pain**

Yes   No

1   2   3   4   5   6   7   8   9   1 0

✳ **Joint pain (knee, wrist, hand, shoulder)**

Yes   No

1   2   3   4   5   6   7   8   9   1 0

✳ **Limited range of motion or function**

Yes   No

1   2   3   4   5   6   7   8   9   1 0

✳ **Muscle soreness, weakness, or cramps**

Yes   No

1   2   3   4   5   6   7   8   9   1 0

✳ **Joint swelling**

Yes   No

1   2   3   4   5   6   7   8   9   1 0

Section subtotal: _____

8. In the last 14 days, have you experienced any of the following mental health symptoms:

✳ **Depression**

Yes   No

1   2   3   4   5   6   7   8   9   1 0

✳ **Nervousness or anxiety**

Yes   No

1   2   3   4   5   6   7   8   9   1 0

✳ **Mood swings (e.g., irritability)**

Yes   No

1   2   3   4   5   6   7   8   9   1 0

✳ **Bingeing, purging, or restrictive eating**

Yes   No

1   2   3   4   5   6   7   8   9   1 0

✳ **Easily distracted or difficulty concentrating (brain fog)**

Yes   No

1   2   3   4   5   6   7   8   9   1 0

Section subtotal: _____

9. If you're a woman, in the last 14 days, have you experienced any of the following reproductive or genital symptoms?

* **Genital discharge**

Yes   No

1   2   3   4   5   6   7   8   9   1 0

* **Genital itch**

Yes   No

1   2   3   4   5   6   7   8   9   1 0

* **Vaginal dryness, hot flashes, or night sweats**

Yes   No

1   2   3   4   5   6   7   8   9   1 0

* **Painful sex**

Yes   No

1   2   3   4   5   6   7   8   9   1 0

* **Irregular, missed, or heavy periods**

Yes   No

1   2   3   4   5   6   7   8   9   1 0

Section subtotal: _____

10. If you're a man, in the last 14 days, have you experienced any of the following reproductive or genital symptoms?

* **Genital itch or discharge**

Yes   No

1   2   3   4   5   6   7   8   9   1 0

* **Low or changes to sex drive**

Yes   No

1   2   3   4   5   6   7   8   9   1 0

✳ **Erectile dysfunction or impotence**

Yes   No

1   2   3   4   5   6   7   8   9   1 0

✳ **Testicular lumps, bumps, or pain**

Yes   No

1   2   3   4   5   6   7   8   9   1 0

✳ **Interrupted urinary stream**

Yes   No

1   2   3   4   5   6   7   8   9   1 0

Section subtotal: _____

11. In the last 14 days, have you had a common cold, flu, fever, or other self-limiting infection like bronchitis or a sinus infection?

    Yes ___ * No ___ * Unsure ___

12. In the last 14 days, have you experienced stress that has been difficult to control, or has negatively impacted your daily activities?

    Yes ___ * No ___ * Unsure ___

- **Find your symptom score:** Add up your answers to the first nine questions, including those about your reproductive health based on your gender. This is your symptom score. If your symptom score is:
  - score < = 22: You feel good.
  - 23 < score < 45: You may have a chronic condition.
  - 46 < score < 67: You most likely have a chronic condition.
  - 68 < score: You have at least one chronic condition, and likely have two or more.

- **What your score means:** Your symptom score is an indicator of how you felt over the past two weeks. Your answers to the last two questions about whether you've been sick or experienced an unusual amount of stress can help ascertain whether your symptoms may be due to an isolated illness or particularly hectic week. If you answered "yes" or "unsure" to either question, think about whether your symptoms might be stemming from an illness or too much stress, which may mean your score isn't reflective of your baseline, or of your average normal. That's why I always recommend completing the symptom index more than once, preferably in another two weeks, and tracking your score over time.

  You feel good: You may have some aches and pains or difficulty falling asleep here and there, but overall, you feel good. Your challenge now is to figure out if this is your baseline or an anomaly simply because you had a great last two weeks. Complete the index again in another two weeks, paying attention to whether the same symptoms or body systems light up, which could indicate a potential hot spot.

  You may have a chronic issue: You feel mostly good, but you may have a chronic issue, whether it's been diagnosed or not. But you may also have had a tough last two weeks because you didn't get enough sleep, worked out too hard in the gym, or were fighting off an illness or enduring some other kind of physical strain. Pay attention to whether several different body systems light up with less severe symptoms or, conversely, whether you're struggling with severe symptoms in just one or two areas.

  You most likely have a chronic issue: Unless you've had a super-rough week or a bad cold or other illness, if your score lands in this range, you are most likely dealing with a chronic condition. If you've already been diagnosed, your condition may not be getting managed properly or may be being perpetuated by what you eat or other choices you make on a daily basis. If you haven't been diagnosed with anything, consider making an appointment with a healthcare provider. To help you and your doctor understand what might be wrong, pay attention to whether lots of body systems are lighting up or if you have just one or two systems with severe symptoms.

You have at least one chronic issue: My heart goes out to anyone in this category, as you really don't feel well. You may have a serious chronic condition or multiple chronic conditions, and if so, they are likely not being managed properly and/or your progress is being thwarted by what you do on a daily basis. When I see patients with this score, it's a sign that we need to intervene, even if they look and act healthy, which many people in this category do.

• **Next steps:** Your score can help you identify whether you may have a chronic condition that needs addressing, but it's not the only assessment that matters. After you determine your score, look at each individual body system (represented by each of the nine numbered questions): If for any of the body areas you ranked two or more of the five symptoms with a severity of 4 or greater, that's a good sign that this particular system is struggling or inflamed. This doesn't necessarily mean you have a disease—that system may be receiving some kind of toxic input, whether it's a prescription drug, a certain food, or simply too much stress.

For each symptom on which you scored a 4 or greater, take these next five steps:

1. **Make an appointment.** A doctor may be able to help get to the bottom of what's going on or at least order diagnostic testing. But don't count on your doctor to solve all your problems or reach the right diagnosis. As we talked about in Chapter One, many conventional doctors aren't trained to identify the cause of symptoms but only to treat those symptoms, and many don't

order the right diagnostic tests, oftentimes because they don't know those tests exist. In Chapter Four, I'll explain which tests you may need based on your symptoms and how to ask your doctor for the right assessments.

2. **Tell a story about each symptom.** Every symptom has a story—and retelling that story can help you get to the bottom of what's going on. Start by trying to identify when you think each symptom first started. Look back over the health biography you completed in Chapter One and try to remember what was happening in your life when you first developed that symptom. Did you move to a different place, have surgery, get sick, start a new job, or change your eating habits for some reason? What was your trigger?

3. **Do some investigative work.** If you're able to tell the story about your symptom, that's great, but if not, don't sweat it— it's possible you may get there with time. Either way, the next step is to investigate what makes your symptom feel better or worse. For example, do you usually experience X symptom only when you eat out or Y symptom when you sleep less, drink wine, or skip the gym? Remember to flip the question around and consider which foods or other daily decisions make the symptom feel better.

In addition to what you eat and the other core actions, like exercise, sleep, and alcohol consumption, certain places, circumstances, or time periods can also make a symptom feel better or worse. For example, are you more likely to experience X symptom when you're at work or at home? When you're social or alone? During the week or on the weekend?

4. **Identify the culprit.** Now that you know a few things about what makes your symptom feel better or worse, it's time to try

to connect the dots and identify why those foods, life actions, places, or time periods may be causing you to feel crappy. For example, if you only get X symptom when you eat out, what food (gluten, dairy, more carbs, more sugar) or drink (wine, beer, hard liquor, soda, coffee) are you consuming at restaurants that you don't usually have at home? Or if you only have Y symptom at work, could it be because you're sitting and staring at a screen for hours on end? Or is it because you eat a different lunch than the one you usually have at home? If you never get Z symptom on the weekends, could it be because you're sleeping more or you're less stressed?

5. **Become your own guinea pig.** If you're able to identify what triggers your symptoms, you can start conducting healthy self-experiments to see what improves the way you feel. In other words, once you know the culprit, you can either remove the culprit or make other changes to your daily life to see if doing so improves your symptoms. For example, if you discover that eating at restaurants where you normally consume a ton of empty carbs makes your symptoms worse, try eliminating empty carbs from your nutrition for the next two weeks, then complete the symptom index again.

The symptom index gives you an incredible opportunity to be present with your feelings and connect with your body in real time. It also empowers you to take control of your own health and which way you want your healthcare to tend toward: being well or waiting to get sick. If you take the time to do the symptom index now and repeat it over time, you should celebrate your success: You are on your way to a State Change.

CHAPTER THREE

What Your Life Is Doing to Your Brain

So this was brain surgery.

I stared at the neurosurgeon's hands as he grasped a scalpel and a cauterizer, delicately removing the walnut-sized tumor from deep inside the patient's brain. The operation was precise and intense, but the surgeon had done it at least a thousand times before, and he seemed entirely at ease chitchatting as he performed the craniotomy, ringed by three medical school students, myself included.

The neurosurgeon was making small talk. "What kind of medicine do you plan to go into?" he asked. While it was difficult to focus on what he was saying as we stared into the patient's skull, we were all used to that question. As third-year med students on rotation, we were expected to answer that question with the same type of medicine practiced by the asking physician—surgery, in this instance—just in case that doctor decided to hand us a coveted residency spot someday. Not everyone played along, though. The thirty-year-old ex-banker on my right spoke up first, saying he had come to Columbia College of Physicians and Surgeons to pursue interventional cardiology but was blown away by surgery and was beginning to change his mind. This was a good hedge. The surgeon nodded.

Next to him was a woman in her late twenties with brown, frizzy hair and glasses. "What about you?" the surgeon asked, gesturing to her.

"I'm planning to go into family medicine," she said.

As he continued to peer through his magnifying glasses into the patient's skull, the surgeon paused, then said matter-of-factly, "Why would you do that? Why would you take a spot at Columbia to go into family medicine?"

This is the kind of rhetorical question you don't answer, so we all stood in silence. Then he moved on to me.

"I'm undecided," I said, "but I've always been looking forward to getting into the OR, so I'm so excited to be here." This, of course, was a lie. I have zero hand-eye coordination and would be doing the world a favor by choosing not to go into any procedural field. I knew this. But I had no intention of putting myself in the line of fire.

In my three years at Columbia, I had already learned that primary care enjoyed little respect in the medical community, especially at large academic research institutions like the one I was attending. Primary care is the least likely to be reimbursed by insurance companies and is thereby one of the least lucrative fields in medicine—one reason why it's treated like the boring bread and butter of healthcare. Despite the fact that primary care is the front line of all care—and where doctors arguably have the greatest potential to prevent a patient's course from healthy to sick—it's still considered less intellectual as well as less heroic than fields like cardiology and surgery. In these specialties, unblocking clogged hearts and excising hard-to-reach tumors are all part of the workday, connected with medical codes that command the highest reimbursement fees.

These stereotypes are reinforced by TV shows like *ER* and *Gray's Anatomy*, where physicians are perpetually rushing down hallways beside stretchers, performing last-minute, death-defying procedures under pressure, and delivering grave, unexpected news. Bizarrely, when I got to med school, the hospital felt pretty low on melodrama and predictable by comparison, but the hierarchy of medical value was still evident to me and everyone else from Day One. We got the message, even if the neurosurgeon hadn't been so blunt about it: *You're not here to go into primary care.*

There's a reason, of course, that most of medicine, along with medical prestige, revolves around saving lives: Stopping people from dying is the essence of healthcare and how the field originally developed centuries ago. A severed limb in war or a lethal infection were the things that took most people out of life until the 1940s, when antibiotics arrived on the scene.

Nowadays, the traumas and diseases we face have changed drastically since World War II, as advances in hygiene, vaccines, technology, and safety standards have significantly reduced the number of traumatic accidents and life-threatening infections. Instead, people are living longer and surviving into the new scourges of our time: heart disease, diabetes, depression, dementia, and cancer.

While conventional healthcare has started to pivot to better address these conditions and what can cause or worsen them, medicine for the most part is still largely oriented around critical care and saving the lives of the sick rather than helping people thrive. In today's health system, we wait until someone gets really sick, and ends up in the hospital needing acute care, before we address their cancer, heart disease, diabetes, or whatever other illness put them there. This backwards way of treatment—sickness before wellness—is causing millions of unnecessary illnesses, surgeries, and hospitalizations, not to mention unnecessary pain and suffering.

Take, for example, the statistic that shows that 230 Americans have a foot or entire leg amputated every single day because they have diabetes that is not being properly managed or treated. But if we focused on preventing diabetes through primary care and educating people to make healthier daily decisions around food, these patients wouldn't need critical care—or have to lose a foot and be disabled for the rest of their lives.

The slowness of the industry to reorient itself to the needs of the twenty-first century is rooted primarily in finances. The insurance industry generously reimburses for expensive procedures, surgeries, and specialty drugs, but not for the time it takes for doctors to address a patient's nutrition or environment, which is often all that's needed to obviate the necessity of these procedures, surgeries, and specialty drugs. For example, insurance companies will pay hundreds of thousands of dollars to a surgeon to rip a vein out of a patient's leg and tie it around his or her heart—otherwise known as bypass surgery—but only $150 to a primary care doctor to take the time to work with that patient to treat his or her heart disease and prevent bypass surgery in the first place. One hundred dollars barely covers office supplies and front-desk staff. This payment structure in primary care has led to a revolving door of ten-to-fifteen-minute visits and strapped family doctors who are also expected to do preventive screenings, referrals, prior authorizations, prescriptions, hours upon hours of administrative work, and urgent care (think colds and flu). We don't have primary care or mental health providers who are paid by the conventional healthcare system to spend time with you and evaluate what could be driving your condition. Instead, the formula for the majority of patients is that you have a fifteen-minute visit, you're given a prescription for a drug, and you're sent out the door.

What this means is that it's up to you to do your own homework to find out what's keeping you at a lower baseline, whether it's how you eat, sleep, move, manage stress, or otherwise live your life every day. Most people, including most of my patients, don't realize that these daily core actions are what's causing them to feel not only physically poor but also mentally and emotionally bad. In short, our core actions greatly influence whether we end up with depression, anxiety, brain fog, ADHD, insomnia, and/or another common mental health condition. If you're not considering how your core actions are affecting your energy and flow, you likely won't be able to solve the mental or emotional issues you have. Moreover, if you don't take the time to assess how your daily actions may be impacting your mood, you may not ever be able to feel as clearheaded, positive, passionate, or joyful as you're capable of feeling.

None of this is to say that taking a few yoga classes or eating more leafy greens will suddenly cure you of clinical depression or anxiety or help you reach a whole new level of happiness. But changing just one toxic input to your mental health can help you reach a new baseline, or a new normal for how you feel on a consistent, daily basis. And this is huge. Enormous. Because if you've grown accustomed to operating at only 60 percent your baseline, you may not realize you're functioning at subpar levels, because subpar has been your norm for so long. This is why completing the PSI at the end of Chapter Two is so important: If you discover you have several high-scoring symptoms, you're most likely operating below your baseline. I also suggest that you think back to the last time you felt well: If the answer is months or even years ago, it's likely a clue that you're living below baseline and are a prime candidate for a breakthrough. In order to have breakthrough, though, you need to change something about your core actions, whether you start exercising most days of the week, for example, identify and eliminate a food allergy, or address a nutritional deficiency. That's how you reach 80 percent or even 90 percent of your baseline, with more energy, clarity, optimism, and even joy than you may have ever thought possible.

Discovering a new baseline is a powerful thing, even if you maintain it only for a short period of time. And if you happen to fall back to your old normal, you'll now know it's a suboptimal way to exist and that more energy, clarity, and optimism are not only attainable but also a much better way to live. You'll also know what you can do to get back to feeling good, because you'll have gotten there before; it's no longer a mystery. You'll know this not only on an intellectual level but also on a visceral level: Your body will be able to feel when you're suboptimal and want to help get you back to full throttle.

To reach a new normal, you first have to figure out which core actions are preventing you from feeling optimal—because you can't manage what you can't measure. This means evaluating the things you do with your body and mind on a daily basis to find out what might be making you more unwell, physically and/or mentally.

In Chapter One, you learned how to tell the story of your health through your health biography (see page 19). In Chapter Two, you identified how you really feel by using the symptom index (see page 32). Now, with this chapter, I want to help you identify the core actions you do every day that may be eroding your mental and emotional health.

The Five Core Actions That Impact Energy and Flow

The things that impact our mental and emotional health the most happen outside a doctor's office. After seeing thousands of patients for years, I know there are five core actions that have the greatest effect on our mood: (1) nutrition, (2) exercise, (3) sleep, (4) technology, and (5) alcohol and drugs.

A few important notes before we dive in. First, I want to recognize that relationships, particularly those with our family, friends, colleagues, and romantic partners, can play a major role in our mental health. Loneliness and lack of community are becoming epidemics in and of themselves. But how we invest in our relationships to improve our mental health is a whole other topic, for a different book. For now, I want to focus on the everyday toxins and decisions that impact us on a physical level.

I also want to recognize that when we get to the alcohol and drug section, there is an important line between use, abuse, and addiction. Alcohol or drug addiction is a disease and not something a person suffering from can simply turn off or make a choice about. What I want to address are common patterns of alcohol and drug misuse and abuse that I see in many of my patients that have yet to become addiction but that are deeply detrimental.

Finally, I want to acknowledge that past traumas and present-day realities, like financial hardship, systemic racism, food deserts, and lack of access to healthcare, can greatly influence our mental health but aren't in our control. In helping thousands of patients who are experiencing or have a history of deep trauma, personal loss, or financial hardship, I know these conditions make it even more imperative that we find out how best to address the core actions, no matter how simple, straightforward, or small, that *are* in the patient's control. In other words, life can be hard. For some of us, it can be really, really hard—and so we need all the help we can get to feel as good as we can in order to face the very real, very big challenges before us. My goal for you is progress, not perfection, and the self-knowledge to live even better than you are today, no matter where you're starting from. So let's dive in.

Food for Energy and Flow

We've all had a sugar rush, a coffee headache, or a bad-oyster GI moment. We know how food can instantly make us feel awful. But what I overlooked in myself for years and now see in my patients all the time is the way in which the foods we eat every day—even the ones we love and that we think are making us feel good—are actually eroding our mental health. I'm not talking about feeling low-energy because you didn't eat enough calories or sleepy because you had a big meal. It's something easier to miss but far more important: What we eat day in and day out is one of the biggest determinants of whether we feel anxious, depressed, foggy, fatigued, irritable, distracted, dissatisfied, or otherwise in a low mood.

If there's one nutritional culprit for low mood above all others, it's sugar. Perhaps the most detrimental way food can influence your energy and mood is if, like most Americans, you eat a diet high in refined sugar, flour, and other carbs. Most of my patients think there's no way they're consuming as much sugar as they are. But sugar is in everything, including many foods labeled "healthy." That's why it's not surprising that the average American consumes nearly sixty pounds of sugar a year—that's three pounds per week, and nearly seventeen teaspoons every day. Think about that for a second: You probably can't imagine swallowing seventeen spoonfuls of sugar in a row. But you're doing just that, every day.

Our sugar habit comes from being surrounded by a sea of packaged, processed convenience foods that have been marketed to us as a "normal" way to eat. These foods include all the obvious offenders like soda, cookies, cakes, breakfast cereals, jams, and other sweet foods and drinks, but also a ton of savory items, too, including protein bars, smoothies, coffee drinks, sports drinks, frozen diet meals, bread, crackers, condiments, gluten-free snacks, sauces, etc. What's more, since half of all the calories the average American consumes come from ultrarefined foods packed with processed carbs, most of what we eat, sweet or not, breaks down into simple sugar anyway, flooding our bodies with even more sweet stuff.

For the record, an ultrarefined food is a processed starch or grain that is dense with additives, preservatives, dyes, and other industrial chemicals. Think "pea crisps" as much as Doritos, sports bars and energy drinks, and any other food that can sit on a shelf in a bag or a box for months or even years. They're often the cheapest, most accessible foods found on store shelves, made from subsidized crops like corn, wheat, and soy, along with industrial dairy products that have led to whey protein and lactose (milk) sugars in everything. These foods are ubiquitous because we've made it economically essential for them to be ubiquitous. And now even the most health-conscious among us, myself included, have a hard time escaping them.

What all this sugar is doing to our mood isn't only incredibly damaging, it's also multifaceted. For starters, too much sugar causes your blood sugar levels to take a daily roller-coaster ride, with a high that makes you feel optimistic and energetic, followed by a low that can leave you irritable, lethargic, anxious, or even angry. We've all felt the crash. But beyond the immediate peaks and valleys we can register, over time sugar also kills the healthy bacteria in your body's digestive tract, also known as the microbiome, that are responsible for making brain chemicals like serotonin and dopamine, referred to as neurotransmitters, that we need for mental and emotional stability. What's more, when eaten regularly, sugar can lead to inflammation throughout the body, including inside the brain, which can create mood conditions like depression—so much so that some researchers have suggested renaming depressive disorders "metabolic syndrome Type II."

Sugar and other refined carbs aren't the only offenders that can give you what my friend Dr. Mark Hyman calls FLC syndrome: Feel Like Crap syndrome. Many of my patients have undiagnosed food sensitivities, intolerances, or outright allergies that they don't know about until we do a deep dive into their overall health by performing diagnostic testing and doing a thorough nutritional assessment. Food sensitivities and intolerances aren't just limited to gluten and dairy but can also occur with less-hyped ingredients like soy, eggs, and corn, which are frequently found in processed foods.

Regardless of which ingredient is the culprit, food intolerances can be detrimental to both your physical *and* mental health. That's because when you eat a food your body doesn't tolerate well, it can lead to immediate allergy symptoms like itching and hives, as well as more subtle symptoms like indigestion, headaches, inflammation, thyroid irregularities, and weight gain, along with brain fog, anxiety, depression, and other mood disorders. These subtler symptoms manifest more slowly and insidiously over time than more obvious allergic reactions, and in ways that are more difficult to pinpoint until you eliminate that food for at least a few weeks.

Food sensitivities can have surprising impacts. In my husband's case, regularly eating gluten-containing products like bread and pasta leads to anger, irritability, and impatience. He has no other symptoms: His gut feels fine, and he doesn't break out or have any joint pain. But if he eats wheat more than once every few weeks, his mood goes haywire. He's experimented multiple times to see if there could be another trigger, but it always comes down to gluten, which likely causes microbial changes in his gut and low-grade brain inflammation that alters the way he sees the world.

One recent Saturday, my husband was extra irritable with me because I didn't give him enough advance notice for a social engagement. I thought back over the past two weeks and realized that we'd been eating more takeout, including some bread, pizza, and scallion pancakes from our favorite local Chinese restaurant, which all added up to a more regular influx of wheat than we normally would have. I reminded him to get strict about his gluten consumption. In less than a week, his mood softened, and we proved again that wheat and refined flour make him irritable.

If you think gluten sensitivities or their effects on our mood aren't real, I can tell you for the sake of my marriage that they are. And for anyone dealing with ongoing depression or anxiety, the addition of brain inflammation and irritability caused by a food insensitivity can make the difference between being able to cope with life and manage positive relationships and not being able to do either.

There's another way your ultrarefined eating habits may be sabotaging your mood. If you're consuming mostly processed and refined foods, like many people do, you may not be getting enough essential nutrients, including omega-3 fats, B vitamins, iron, vitamin D, and magnesium, along with antioxidants and phytonutrients found in whole plants. Combined, these nutrients work to lower inflammation in the brain and boost mood and mental health in a number of ways.

For example, not getting enough "marine" omega-3 fats, so called because they're found primarily in fatty fish, can trigger or worsen mood issues, since they help the body build cell membranes; without enough of them, your brain's neural growth and neuroplasticity—i.e., its ability to change and reorganize itself to process stress and new information—can be slowed. B vitamins, such as B_{12}, found in animal foods (like beef, fish, and dairy) and folate (B_9) found in plant foods (like beans, lentils, and leafy greens), are necessary to make neurotransmitters like serotonin—which is why studies have shown that being low in Bs can put you at a higher risk for depression and anxiety. And being low in these nutrients is also super-common: Surveys estimate up to 40 percent of Americans may be short in B_{12}, while 95 percent of all Americans don't meet the estimated average for omega-3s.

Exercise for Energy and Flow

If you're not moving in a way that gets your heart pumping, your muscles ripping, and your sweat pouring on a regular basis, the hard truth is that you can't expect to feel good, mentally or emotionally. It's really that simple. Doing some form of exercise, whether it's a traditional workout like running or yoga or something more unconventional like gardening or dancing, isn't a *nice-to-have* for your mental health: It's a *must-have*.

Here's the deal: The human body wasn't meant to sit for hours on end, even though that's what we now do on a daily basis. The average office worker sits for up to fifteen hours per day, a habit that can not only lead to weight gain, obesity, and other chronic physical conditions but also impair mental and emotional stability. That's because sitting all day slows blood and oxygen flow to the brain, driving up inflammation that can cause poor mood.

Moving your body, on the other hand, has been shown to lower inflammation, produce feel-good endorphins, and give your mind a physical outlet for any anxiety or stress you may be suffering. Studies also show that physical activity can cause the brain to grow new neurons and, over time, rewire neural pathways that help stabilize mood and emotions. There's something else about exercise that often gets overlooked when we talk about physical activity and mental health. When you mix low activity levels with a high-sugar diet—a common combo for most people—the union is like kryptonite for our minds and mood, leading to poor sleep, low-grade panic attacks, and depression. I see this all the time in patients. In some instances, they have no other drivers for a mood disorder other than that they're sitting too much and consuming too much sugar, a combination that many human minds simply can't withstand after years on end. Think of it like a house in a storm: If your house weathered a tropical storm for a day or two, it would probably be fine. If your house was battered by a tropical storm for two straight years, the roof might leak, the basement would probably flood, and the siding would come off. Similarly, humans aren't meant to live in a permanent tropical storm of sitting and sugar.

It often surprises my patients when I show them the studies demonstrating that exercise has been proven to be just as effective as some antidepressants in treating mood disorders. One study from researchers at Duke University, for example, found that people who did some type of aerobic exercise regularly for four months experienced an equivalent reduction in depression to those who took Zoloft for the same time period. More interestingly, the exercise-only group was much less likely than those taking Zoloft to relapse with depressive symptoms after six months. That's not to say a long run is going to instantly alleviate your anxiety or depression. But if you have mood problems or simply don't feel as clear, positive, or passionate as you want, you're missing out on a powerful antidote by not moving your body on a regular basis. For most people, exercise isn't strictly about getting a better bikini body or becoming an athlete but about doing something on a daily or near-daily basis that can help them feel better and better about themselves in every way.

Technology for Energy and Flow

I'm willing to bet no medical professional has ever talked with you about whether your relationship with your phone is harming your mental health. While some people may be aware of the danger, most don't actively consider how all the hours they spend on computers, smartphones, and social media may be influencing their mood. But the truth is, modern technology has changed our brains—for the worse.

As we spend more time with screens today than we ever have before, with some reports showing the average American stares at a device up to seventeen hours per day, the negative effects of too much tech have really started to reveal themselves, prompting even former executives of Facebook to sound the alarm about what our tech obsession is doing to our brains.

There are several reasons why tech is eroding our mental and emotional health. Research shows that both our mobile devices and social media accounts are as addictive as street drugs, stimulating the same neural pathways as cocaine, making it nearly impossible to put down our phones and stop checking our Insta. Like most addictions, the one to technology is isolating us from our friends and families and preventing us from engaging in real-life activities like exercising, cooking, reading, and all the other pursuits that can bring people calm and joy.

While you may think your computer, phone, or social media feed is providing you with some calm or joy—or at least some entertainment—studies show tech actually accomplishes just the opposite. The hours we spend on Instagram and TikTok cause us to compare ourselves to others, fueling feelings of inadequacy, low self-esteem, loneliness, anxiety, and depression. This is part of the reason why teen suicide rates skyrocketed after smartphones become popular, as kids have stayed within arm's reach of their social media and the anxiety and low self-esteem social media fuels.

Even if you're rarely on social media, there's another way your phone and computer may be impairing your mental health and mood: Tech is literally turning our brains into mush due to all the time we spend staring at screens, regardless of what we're doing when we look at them. Similar to street drugs, technology can shrink your brain's gray matter, impair white matter function, reduce cortical thickness, drive up cravings, and limit overall cognitive function (we'll detail how these detriments can actually occur in Chapter Seven). You don't need to be a neuroscientist to know these effects can harm your mental health, reducing cognitive capacity and sapping mental and emotional stability.

Staring at screens all day can create problems in the other areas of your life, too. You don't move much when you consume technology, for example—which is one reason why Americans sit more now than they did before the advent of smartphones, laptops, tablets, gaming consoles, and other gizmos and gadgets.

Another issue with tech use is that screens emit damaging blue light, which interferes with the body's production of the sleep hormone melatonin, disrupting your ability to fall asleep or stay asleep.

Finally, all our personal technology is making it impossible for any of us to relax. You likely already know something about the body's fight-or-flight response, instigated whenever we're faced with a stressful or potentially dangerous situation. Back in our ancient ancestors' day, this danger could be a hungry lion or hostile tribe. Today, though, we're in a continual standoff with a mound of emails, a barrage of distressing online news, and accumulating social media feeds, all of which keep us in a constant state of stimulation. While we may not feel the same sense of fear our ancestors did when they saw a snarling lion, we still create stress hormones and other chemicals that ratchet up our anxiety and stress levels. No wonder we all feel exhausted at the end of the day, even when we've done nothing for hours but sit in our chairs and stare at our screens.

Sleep for Energy and Flow

You already know what happens if you don't get a good night's sleep: You feel like crap the next day. We all do. But when you do this night after night, the ramifications exceed a little lethargy, some unsightly eye bags, and maybe a less-than-ideal job on that work report. There are multiple ways you can suffer from prolonged sleep deprivation. The most obvious way is that you're simply not getting enough sleep, meaning you average less than seven hours per night. But even if you clock seven hours or more, you could still be sleep-deprived if the time you spend in bed isn't actually high-quality or restful sleep, meaning you're not averaging enough time in deep sleep cycles. Your sleep quality can also be jeopardized if you're using medications like zolpidem (Ambien), which don't allow your body to experience a complete sleep cycle and can worsen and even cause anxiety, depression, brain fog, and other mental health problems.

One reason inadequate sleep wreaks havoc on mood and mental health is that sleep is literally when your brain takes out its trash, clearing neurotoxins and other cognitive debris that accumulate during the day. If you don't give your brain this critical time to clean itself, brain trash (made up of the chemical by-products of our metabolism) builds up and your mind begins to malfunction, making you more vulnerable to cognitive ailments like Alzheimer's, along with mental and emotional instability.

Sleep is also when the human brain processes emotions. If you're not getting enough restorative rest for whatever reason, unprocessed emotions can overpower you during the day. Without enough sleep, your amygdala, an almond-sized mass in the brain that helps regulate emotions, starts working overtime to try to regain control. The result is that your brain can't discern between a crisis and an event that isn't such a big deal, causing you to overreact and feel irritability, anger, negativity, confusion, sadness, and other unpleasant emotions.

There are two other outcomes I see in my patients who don't sleep well. Since they're not getting enough restorative rest, they start a rinse-and-repeat cycle of caffeine and sugar to wake them up during the day, bookended by alcohol or sleeping pills to help them unwind at night. The problem is that this cycle only worsens their ability to get any kind of restorative rest, while all that coffee, sugar, booze, and/or sleeping pills intensifies their mood issues. Because lack of sleep is also associated with low-grade cognitive dysfunction, they also don't make good decisions the next day when they haven't slept well, making them more vulnerable to negativity, low self-esteem, and other problem emotions.

If you wake up in the morning and still don't feel rested, you may also have a sleep disorder, like sleep apnea, that's interfering with your body's ability to complete all the necessary stages of sleep. This isn't your fault, but it's something that should be investigated and treated. Stress, physical inflammation, and blood sugar problems can also interfere with your sleep quality even if you're averaging seven hours per night or more.

Whatever way you look at it, not getting enough restorative sleep can leave you stuck in permanent "meh" mode. When we don't feel rested, our inability to cope with our emotions goes sideways and things look foggier, fuzzier, more stressful, anxious, dark, and sometimes even downright depressing.

Substance Misuse and Abuse for Energy and Flow

There's a reason I specify substance *misuse* and *abuse* here rather than *addiction*. If you know or believe you're an alcoholic or have a genuine addiction to other drugs, you probably have some idea of the damage you're already doing to your mind and mood. Either way, don't go it alone: No matter how many times you've tried to get help, there is a doctor, psychiatrist, psychologist, 12-step program, or detox center that can help you beat addiction. As I said at the beginning of this chapter, addiction is a disease, not a habit.

The issue I want to address here is that the majority of Americans (and the majority of my patients) aren't clinically addicted to substances but drink alcohol, smoke weed, or take recreational drugs on a semi-regular or regular basis in a way that depletes their mental health. While I believe there's a level of occasional consumption of alcohol, marijuana, and even psychedelic drugs like ketamine and psilocybin that can be healthy and even supportive of a positive mental state, the fact is that I rarely see anyone using these substances successfully at a healthy level.

Truth time: I personally enjoy a glass of wine a couple of nights a week or the occasional cocktail at dinner. A joint is, for me, a once-in-a-blue thing, although I honestly wish I liked marijuana better, because I think a dosing pen that filters smoke can be a healthy way to relax. But there's a big difference between using alcohol or marijuana to feel even better when you already feel good and relying on substances as the only way to maintain a baseline of stability or to keep anxiety away, which is what I see most people doing. It's the "just get me to the end of the day so I can have my glass of wine/joint" mode that's the problem. This is when you know the substance is making up for a deficiency in baseline happiness.

In my patients, I see something I call a pre-addiction phase that comes before outright addiction, where they're drinking alcohol or consuming pot as a way to cope with stress, sadness, emptiness, general anxiety, social anxiety, or other unpleasant emotions. Alcohol or weed is their primary way of feeling good, dealing with stress, *and* socializing, and they end up ingesting a steady drip of booze or inhale of pot to accomplish all three. This is different than a substance addiction, which I define as a disease or biochemical dependency that's outside of someone's control. What I'm talking about here is substance habituation, meaning you use substances out of habit, for how they make you feel, which can eventually lead to biochemical dependency.

This is common, and most patients don't think it's a problem—they simply don't make the link between their substance use and their mental state. But then they do a mini-detox, and they're shocked to discover they feel so much better, physically and emotionally, without a continual stream of narcotics into their bloodstream. They begin to realize that, while alcohol or pot hasn't derailed their relationships, careers, or general ability to get through life, their continual use is eroding their ability to live *happily*.

While alcohol may be sanctified in our society as both a coping mechanism and a social necessity, it actually doesn't do the job in either application: Booze is a depressant that reduces the brain's ability to process emotions, feel aroused, and be socially stimulated. More so, drinking on a regular basis, even if you aren't addicted, can cause or worsen anxiety and depression. Alcohol interferes with sleep, preventing the kind of deep sleep we need to feel rested and restored.

Pot has its own problems: While some weed may be okay in moderation, research shows daily use can be the direct cause of anxiety, depression, and other mood disorders.

Whether you use weed, alcohol, or even sugar to feel good, these substances, when habitual, replace your body's natural ability to regulate your mood. In other words, when you rely on substances to improve your mood, you disrupt your body's own capability to feel good, eventually sabotaging its ability to reset itself and find energy and flow.

*

If you've read this list of core actions and are thinking, *F&^%, I have to completely overhaul my life*, don't worry: you don't. And you certainly don't have to do it all at once. I know it's not easy to change how you eat, move, sleep, and do the other core actions I've listed here. Whether we're aware of it or not, most of us are resistant to altering what we do on a daily basis, myself included.

I'm a mom of three kids, for example, and I've recently let exercise fall mostly by the wayside, despite the fact that I feel calmer, sleep better, and see the world more positively after I use an elliptical, take a yoga class, or go for a long walk. But I know exercise is just one of the tools that I have in my biohacker's toolkit that will help me generate happiness, even if being active takes effort and goes against the grain of what my day as a doctor, mom, and business owner dictates, which is to stay sedentary. But when you have your own tools and know what they can do for your mood, sometimes you have to ignore the doubters and lemmings, psych yourself up, and biohack your way to better health.

For example, I know I can choose just one of my tools and start exercising more, drop the sugar or gluten, or get a few hours away from my phone. With any of those changes, I can reach a new baseline where I feel 5 percent better—enough to keep me using my tools until I feel 10 percent better, then 20 percent better, and so on. In other words, a little bit of action goes a long way.

Another reason you don't have to change everything at once: While we've looked at nutrition, exercise, sleep, tech, and substance abuse in isolation, they're all interrelated. When you sleep poorly, for example, you're less likely to exercise and more likely to have sugar cravings and make bad food choices. When you drink alcohol, you're more likely to eat unhealthy food, blow off the gym, and get a poor night's sleep. When you stare at screens all day, you move less and may consume more processed convenience food, as most of us do when we spend much of our waking hours gazing at computers, smartphones, or TVs. Eating too much sugar makes it difficult to get restorative rest and can leave you feeling so anxious, irritable, or lethargic that nothing sounds better than having a drink while scrolling through social media. You get the point.

Because core actions are all interrelated, you don't have to act on all five at once—or even more than one at a time—to see results for your mood. I tell my patients that if they can change just one core action at a time, they'll likely influence a few others naturally, without even trying. If you start exercising, for example, you'll have less time for tech, improve your ability to get a good night's sleep, help your body balance blood sugar, and be more motivated to make healthier food choices during the day. If you take a two-week break from booze, you'll sleep better, eat better, and find yourself more likely to exercise. In short, you don't have to overhaul your entire life: You can reach a new baseline simply by changing one core action at a time. But to get the most bang for your buck, you need to pinpoint which action is going to have the biggest impact right off the bat.

Identifying the Core Action That's Impacting Your Mental Health the Most

At Parsley, we do an in-depth social analysis of all our new patients, which means we take the time to look at how they're living their lives beyond what symptoms or prior medical history they have. We do this because we know that getting someone to change how they eat, move, or manage stress may be the true unlock they need to help heal a chronic ailment or illness.

We want to know not only what you're eating in an average week but also how often you cook at home, whether you read nutritional labels, how the other people in your household eat, if you snack in the middle of the night, whether you travel often, if you weigh yourself, and what foods you don't like. We do the same deep dive into your exercise, sleep, tech consumption, and substance use habits, in addition to assessing your stress level and where you think your tension is coming from. As one of our patients recently tweeted, "I've never felt more *seen* than by the Parsley Health intake questionnaire."

The reason we ask all these questions, which I can guarantee no other doctor has ever asked you before, is that we can do all the diagnostic testing in the world, but if one or more of your core life actions is either worsening or causing a physical, mental, or emotional issue, we may not be able to get to the bottom of what's going on and help you lift whatever's blocking your ability to heal.

Parsley's full intake form would be too long to include in this book, but I've simplified it here into a quick and dirty but still super-insightful self-assessment that will help you identify the primary core action amplifying your depression, causing your brain fog, worsening your fatigue, or driving your chronic illness. The goal here is to get a hot take on which area of your daily life you should focus on first to make changes. Then, since healthy habits usually snowball, you can take advantage of the snowball effect to feel better faster.

In the following self-assessment, circle the degree of regularity for which you do what's described in each statement. Take your time and try to answer the questions as honestly as you can. I recommend completing the exercise alone in a quiet place where you can be truthful with yourself. Oftentimes, the biggest blocker in creating our own State Change is accepting which daily actions aren't serving us, even if they feel essential to the way we live.

1. I eat refined foods like pasta, crackers, bread, cookies, chips, cakes, sweets, bars, sodas, sports drinks, juices, or foods that come out of a sealed plastic wrapping every day or every other day (note: this includes all pasta, crackers, bread, etc., regardless of whether it's gluten-free, grain-free, vegan, or all-organic): Never, Sometimes, Mostly, Always

2. I am sedentary (no workouts or exercise) most days of the week: Never, Sometimes, Mostly, Always

3. I get less than seven to eight hours of restful, unaided sleep every night, without using medication to fall asleep: Never, Sometimes, Mostly, Always

4. I spend at least five hours a day looking at a computer or phone screen: Never, Sometimes, Mostly, Always

5. I drink alcohol, smoke weed, or use other recreational drugs more days than I don't: Never, Sometimes, Mostly, Always

6. I feel stressed on a daily or weekly basis: Never, Sometimes, Mostly, Always

7. I exercise, meditate, read a book, spend time in nature, or sober socialize as a way to feel good: Never, Sometimes, Mostly, Always

8. I feel supported by my friends, family, and/or chosen family: Never, Sometimes, Mostly, Always

If you answered "Mostly" or "Always" to questions 1–5, you have at least one toxic core action that's making it harder for you to generate happiness, manage depression and anxiety, heal from trauma, or beat brain fog.

If you answered "Sometimes" to any question 1–5, one of these core actions may be the Achilles' heel that's preventing you from feeling much better than you do now.

If you answered "Mostly" or "Always" to question 6 or "Never" or "Sometimes" to questions 7 and 8, you may have identified ways in which your regular environment is impeding your ability to improve or address the toxic inputs you discovered you're coping with in questions 1–5. For example, chronic stress or lack of social support could be driving you to eat poorly, consume too much media, or turn to alcohol.

After you've analyzed your answers, pick one—and only one—core action to address that you assessed was a factor in questions 1–5, whether that's how you eat, how you move, how you sleep, your tech habits, or your substance use. If your self-assessment shows you have more than one problematic core action, pick the one that you believe will be easiest for you to change. This will set you up for success and help you begin to take baby steps toward overhauling your other core actions with the healthy snowball effect we discussed earlier. Going forward in this book, keep your most problematic core action(s) in mind as we cover how to overhaul each one step-by-step, helping you develop a real biohacker's toolkit to accomplish your very own State Change.

CHAPTER FOUR

The Diagnostic Tests You Really Need

*I*t's not in my head. It's not in my head.

It was all Sam could think as she picked up her purse and tried to manage a smile for her doctor. Was that obliging pity that she saw? Sam's physician looked back at her as though she were a sweet old lady who was a delusional hypochondriac. Sam nodded back and walked out of the office and to her Honda Civic, making sure to steer the car well out of the parking lot before bursting into tears.

The thing is, Sam wasn't delusional or even old: She was a forty-seven-year-old woman who was constantly tired, so much so that she felt fatigued after sleeping eight or even ten hours a night—or trying to sleep, at least. She had gained more than fifteen pounds in the last year, never felt like she could concentrate, and would feel so sad at times that she'd frequently deteriorate into a crying jag for no apparent reason—and not just because her doctor had told her her symptoms were just in her head.

That prognosis—"it's in your head"—was her doctor's best bet for why Sam was experiencing fatigue, brain fog, and weight gain after forty-six years of a relatively healthy relationship between her brain and body. Or maybe, Sam's doctor hypothesized, she was doing too much—at that point, Sam was working full-time while studying to earn her master's degree in education. Or maybe it was just a funk? Also, Sam's doctor added, *This is sometimes what happens when you get older.*

Old?! Sam thought, as her sadness turned to anger inside her Civic. *I'm only forty-seven! I'm too young to be that old!* But as she continued to drive through St. Louis to her home, where her two kids, two cats, and one husband were all waiting to be fed, Sam began to have a change of heart. Maybe her fatigue and brain fog *were* all in her head. Maybe she was depressed. Maybe she was even crazy! Or maybe she just needed to sleep more (was that possible?), eat less, or go on an antidepressant.

Maybe.

Or maybe Sam just needed to see a doctor who was willing to take her symptoms seriously and had the time, desire, and expertise to get to the bottom of what was really going on with Sam's health.

In Sam's case, she knew something was wrong, but she had been taught to listen to doctors and, in general, to ignore herself until things got really bad. But now, things had gotten so bad that she felt like she wasn't even herself. She hadn't always felt like this—after all, it wasn't like she had been perpetually tired since she was a child—and she'd only become super-fatigued about a year or so ago. Sam didn't think it was entirely in her head, and there was no reason for her suddenly to be depressed, so after doing a few Google searches and reading many blog posts, she signed up to see me at Parsley.

When I met Sam, the first thing I wanted to do was to hear her story—because, as I've shared, the story of your health is the story of your life (see page 18). She told me how she'd gone through a major stressor several years ago after her husband lost his job. She started working longer hours to compensate, and even though she was officially still the family cook, she started serving and eating a lot of frozen dinners to save time. Over the year, her symptoms worsened, which she originally chalked up to stress. But she didn't feel that stressed—or, really, the most stressful thing was what was happening to her body.

As a doctor, I knew it could definitely be a lot more than stress. I knew that Sam could have a thyroid disorder, an adrenal problem, a blood sugar imbalance, a nutrient deficiency, an autoimmune condition, or a gut issue. All these underlying conditions are common and treatable, but they have to be identified first in order to be treated.

Yet Sam's primary care doctor had never tested her for any of these conditions. This isn't because Sam's doctor didn't care or wasn't competent: It's because the diagnostic testing for these common conditions isn't today's standard care—especially for women, 20 percent of whom report feeling ignored or dismissed by their healthcare provider. Not only do most doctors fail to run these tests, many also don't know why some of these tests are relevant in the first place, or they wait to do thorough testing until a patient's symptoms have progressed to the point where they feel sick or have already developed a chronic disease.

But at Parsley, I order almost all the diagnostic tests you'll read about in this chapter for every new patient immediately, right after their first visit. I don't do this to show patients we're willing to pull out all the stops for their health: I do it because testing is one of the most important things any doctor can do for your health. Modern diagnostic testing allows us to establish a baseline for your body, mind, and mood that we can track and monitor, showing us whether and where you're improving and what's driving those positive changes. More important, testing allows us to catch problems before they turn into troubling symptoms or even outright disease. Most often, chronic illness will show up in thorough testing before a patient ever manifests symptoms. And, as in Sam's case, testing allows us to figure out whether there's a physical reason a patient is dealing with fatigue, weight gain, depression, burnout, or other super-common symptoms, all of which can indicate an underlying condition.

When we tested Sam for more than just the basics, we discovered what we had both suspected all along: Her symptoms weren't in her head. Instead, she had an autoimmune condition, called Hashimoto's thyroiditis, that was causing her to gain weight and feel fatigued, depressed, and foggy. She didn't need to eat less, get more sleep, or take an antidepressant; she needed medication to manage her Hashimoto's, to avoid foods like wheat (which can aggravate the condition), to support her thyroid with certain nutrients so it could function better, and to make other simple changes to her daily actions in order to manage the disease that had disrupted her life. The hack had been there all along for Sam to overhaul her mental health—and it all started with a simple blood test.

Sam's story isn't unique or a one-off outlier that can be chalked up to bad luck or unfortunate circumstances. The vast majority of people with a thyroid disease—60 percent—don't know they have one. That's not because they don't have any symptoms: Most people with thyroid conditions experience many of the same unpleasant problems that Sam did, including weight gain, fatigue, depression, and brain fog.

Thyroid conditions also don't go undiagnosed because the testing is expensive, difficult to do, or invasive. Quite the opposite: A full thyroid panel is really easy to order. A doctor just has to check some boxes, then you can go get a single blood draw, and voila: You have answers that can change your life if your results show that you have Hashimoto's thyroiditis or general hypothyroidism, which means your thyroid isn't functioning properly.

There's so much you can learn about your health and why you might be living below your optimal baseline by taking the time to have some simple diagnostic tests done. If you wait until high inflammation levels show up as joint pain, brain fog, or even heart disease, you're missing the point of modern medicine. Of course, testing requires a trip to the doctor—and I do recommend seeing a functional or integrative doctor. Both receive the same amount of training as conventional physicians do but adopt a more holistic approach to treating the body, not just its symptoms, and usually have more experience ordering comprehensive testing and interpreting the results.

Keep in mind, though, that you didn't develop symptoms overnight, so you can't expect to get rid of them as quickly either. Testing is the first step in a process of discovery and subsequent treatment, but one worth doing: It's the only way to know what you're dealing with in your own body and to identify possible root causes of vague symptoms like fatigue, weight gain, anxiety, brain fog, and even depression, all of which some practitioners dismiss since these symptoms can be not only vague but multifaceted and difficult to diagnose or treat. Testing gives you the hard facts that can help you get on a different treatment trajectory that can change your life.

This is exactly what happened with Sam. But why didn't her doctor discover earlier that she had Hashimoto's? Here's the thing: Most doctors don't order a full thyroid panel that can show Hashimoto's or even hypothyroidism, a common condition that occurs when your thyroid makes too much hormone, which affects one in eight women (although this number is likely higher, since many cases of thyroid disease go undiagnosed due to the lack of testing that we're talking about here).

It's not just thyroid issues, either: Most doctors also don't order simple tests that can identify adrenal fatigue, imbalanced estrogen or testosterone levels, early blood sugar issues, genetic variants, autoimmune disorders, or gastrointestinal conditions. Instead, they tell patients that the hallmark symptoms they're having, like depression, brain fog, anxiety, and fatigue, are in their head or something only a psychiatrist can deal with.

I'm not trying to throw shade on your primary care doctor. She may be a fantastic physician, well meaning, and doing all the basics. After all, the basics are what most primary care doctors are trained to do, what they get paid for, and what they have time for.

I know from experience. When I started seeing patients in residency at a top hospital, we were given only fifteen minutes with every person to cover those basics, which is barely enough time to assess someone's vital signs and refill their medications, let alone begin to peel back the layers to figure out why they might be feeling the way they do. We weren't encouraged or rewarded for putting the puzzle pieces of a person's health story together. Instead, we were trained to zero in on the most pressing problem that day and to do what we needed to do to make sure that person didn't die from that problem. Our process was streamlined down to three steps: Conduct a basic physical exam (which doesn't capture mental health), run basic blood work, and prescribe medication. From there, everything else could be handled by a specialist—if it got so bad as to warrant seeing one.

The basic blood work I was taught to order actually reveals very little about your health, other than your cholesterol, blood sugar, blood cell counts, and whether you might be suffering from an infection. These are all markers that primary care doctors know how to handle, showing them whether a patient might have anemia, diabetes, or signs of heart disease.

But there are so many more things that could be wrong with your health, obviously—and these conditions are getting missed all the time because their associated symptoms, like weight gain, brain fog, and fatigue, aren't life-threatening, and the work to identify and treat them requires a little more effort and investigation than most conventional doctors have the time or training for. When I was in med school, for example, we were told to test only for the bare minimum and then wait for a condition to "declare" itself before we started pulling out all the stops to find out what was really going on.

But I don't think anyone should have to wait to get seriously sick or hospitalized before we test them for the common and treatable health issues that may be causing them to feel awful, physically *or* mentally. As a doctor, I believe in being proactive about your health and actually helping you get and feel better, whether you have an obvious condition like an infection or a slow-moving underlying disorder like an autoimmune disease. That's why we run almost all the tests in this chapter on Day One for every new patient, regardless of what symptoms someone has or doesn't have. Oftentimes, what we discover is that an underlying condition is actually causing mental health issues or making it impossible for someone to work through them with a therapist and/or medication, long before that condition has become a life-threatening disease.

Discovering that a physical condition has been causing you to feel depressed, fatigued, scatterbrained, anxious, and/or foggy can be a giant unlock—oftentimes for both you and your therapist. I once got an email from a New York City psychiatrist thanking me for ordering a test for one of his patients that showed she had blood sugar issues and hormonal imbalances. We had treated those issues with supplements and food changes, and several months later the psychiatrist told me that her depression and extreme fatigue had receded considerably. He was awestruck, because he had been working with her for years and had never once considered that a physical condition was impeding her progress. I held back from reminding him that he had gone to med school and could have ordered those tests. *Happy to help!* I responded instead.

This is why I think everyone should get most of the tests outlined in this chapter every year, regardless of what your symptoms are. This may sound radical, and it is compared to how conventional medicine works. But over and over again, I see conventional medicine using basic blood work as a reactive move, not a proactive one, which fails patients who don't have immediately life-threatening physical, mental, and emotional symptoms caused by underlying conditions.

You can easily take the diagnostic test cheat sheet I've included on pages 91–92 to your primary care doctor and ask that he or she order all of them for you. But if you have the ability and access, I strongly recommend finding a functional- or holistic-medicine doctor. Some tests in this chapter don't identify a specific disease but assess whether your body is functioning suboptimally or is on its way to developing a more severe disease. The results of these tests require expertise to interpret, and if you are functioning below baseline, the solution is usually never as straightforward as a prescription drug—which is why you want someone with a holistic background to help you make certain which core life actions you need to change to get better.

It's ultimately up to you to take control of your health and how you feel, which means putting in the time and effort to find the right doctor or raising your hand with your own primary care physician to make sure you get the right tests. While being your own healthcare advocate and telling your doctor what to do can feel scary at first, it's an empowering move: The power to feel good is in your hands.

Is It My Hormones? Let's Start with Hormone Testing

At Parsley, we test for three different types of hormones in our patients every year: thyroid, adrenal, and sex, including estrogen, progesterone, and testosterone. Since all are distinct, and off levels can indicate different problems, I'll cover each separately.

Thyroid

The thyroid is a butterfly-shaped gland inside your neck that acts like the proverbial foot on the gas pedal of your metabolism. Your thyroid regulates your energy levels, helps your body burn calories, plays a role in your sleep, supports your immune system, and keeps your digestion moving. When your thyroid doesn't produce enough hormones, a condition known as hypothyroidism, you can experience weight gain, depression, and fatigue, along with constipation, sleeping troubles, and low mood.

Today, one in eight women is diagnosed with a thyroid disorder during her lifetime. Thyroid conditions have become more common as Americans consume more ultrarefined foods high in sugar, which interferes with thyroid hormone production. Fueling up on a high-calorie, low-nutrient diet, like most of us do, also keeps people from getting the micronutrients the thyroid needs for optimal function, including selenium, zinc, iodine, and magnesium.

Some chemicals in our food, personal care products, and environment—found in everything from coffee (which can contain concentrated levels of chemical fertilizers and pesticides) to body lotions (most of which have phthalates) to vegetables (which can contain pesticides used in growing)—are also hormone disruptors, blocking the thyroid's ability to do its job. While your body may produce enough hormones, these toxins prevent those hormones from doing their job at the cellular level, tricking your brain into thinking you need more hormones and triggering your body to produce more, all to no avail.

Some autoimmune disorders can result in your immune system attacking your thyroid gland. We'll talk more about those conditions on page 81, and testing for inflammation and immune markers, but if you're suffering from an autoimmune disorder and don't know it, your thyroid may be paying the price.

Add up all the ways to develop an underactive or fully dysfunctional thyroid, and holy cow: no wonder that thyroid conditions are so common. That's why it's confounding to know that most conventional doctors don't regularly screen for thyroid disorders—or if they do, they're running a basic thyroid panel, which won't pick up all the possible problems with the gland. If you tell your doctor you suspect you might have a thyroid issue, he or she will likely test only your levels of thyroid-stimulating hormone (TSH). If your TSH levels are high, it means you're not producing enough thyroid hormones and have hypothyroidism.

While the test may sound cut-and-dried, it's not. First, there's a rather wide range of "normal" for TSH, anywhere between 0.5 mlU/L and 5.0 mlU/L. So if your TSH clocks in at 4 mlU/L or even 4.9 mlU/L, your doctor may tell you that you're "fine" when your thyroid is not functioning optimally at all. I consider TSH levels between 0.2 and 3.0 mlU/L to be optimal and up to 3.5 mlU/L to be acceptable if a patient is asymptomatic. But a result of 3.5 mlU/L or over signifies to me that your thyroid is stressed or struggling.

Second, and more important, TSH levels provide only a narrow and incomplete picture of thyroid function. Just because your body produces enough thyroid hormone doesn't mean it's able to use it. The body needs to convert the thyroid hormone free thyroxine, or T4, into triiodothyronine (T3) in order for it to do its job in your cells. If you don't have enough T4 or T3, you'll have hypothyroidism even if your TSH levels are fantastic.

A simple TSH test also won't show whether you might have Hashimoto's thyroiditis or Graves's disease, both of which are autoimmune disorders that cause hypothyroidism or hyperthyroidism, respectively, by triggering the immune system to attack the gland. That's why I always test for thyroid antibodies by screening for thyroid peroxidase (TPO) and antithyroglobulin antibodies, both which can show whether someone may have Hashimoto's. For Graves's, I test only if someone shows specific symptoms like weight loss, diarrhea, or tremors in their hands or fingers, since Graves's is much more rare to see.

I see so many people, especially women (but men, too), whose mood issues and burnout are either being worsened by undiagnosed thyroid disorders or else it's their thyroid that's causing them to feel crappy in the first place. Many are taking antidepressants and not getting any better—and they won't, until we treat their thyroid condition. We can do this with medication, but sometimes all it takes is making a few specific changes to your nutrition or toxin exposure. Either way, there are easy hacks that can overhaul your health and even reverse a mood disorder that you've been dealing with for years.

Adrenal

Adrenal health is gaining more traction among doctors, especially in the functional and holistic space, as we develop more accurate testing and a better understanding for how the adrenals affect physical and mental health. The adrenals are small glands, one of which sits over each of the kidneys like a little hat. They help make certain hormones, like cortisol—the body's stress hormone—along with key neurotransmitters like epinephrine, otherwise known as adrenaline, which stimulates the body's fight-or-flight response.

The adrenals don't have a mind of their own: They produce hormones like cortisol and neurotransmitters like epinephrine when your brain tells them to.

So, if you encounter a lion in the jungle or get mugged on the street, your brain will signal your adrenals to start pumping out these chemicals. This worked really well when human beings had to deal with only periodic, punctuated moments of stress. But in today's modern world, we now face stress from the moment we get up to the time we go to sleep, as we're barraged by work, media, family, social obligations, and urban or suburban existence, without any nature or peace and quiet to calm us down. Some people try to fight this stress with exercise, but today's trend of super-intense workouts, like CrossFit or spinning classes with screaming instructors and ear-splitting music, can sometimes only ratchet up our tension levels.

What all of this has created is a society where most of us are always hyped up and stressed out, with no healthy balance between stimulation and downtime. Our adrenals are nearly always pumping out cortisol and epinephrine, and over time, they can stop functioning properly, producing these chemicals at the wrong times or in too low amounts. This doesn't mean you have a disease but rather a functional disorder—something conventional doctors have a difficult time diagnosing or even understanding.

At Parsley, we check adrenal function by asking patients to collect urine or saliva samples at different intervals during the day, which we then analyze for cortisol and related breakdown compounds, like cortisone. Your cortisol levels fluctuate naturally throughout the day—they're higher in the morning to help you get up and go, and lower at night to help you wind down and sleep. But if your cortisol remains elevated all day or is too low in the morning, something may be functionally wrong with your adrenals.

I see people with various forms of adrenal fatigue all the time. I have a patient in his late thirties, for example, who has a high-stress job. When he first came to see me, he was drinking a ton of coffee and barely sleeping. He was also getting sick with colds and other low-grade infections all the time. He had acute anxiety, was making irrational decisions, and would often erupt in angry outbursts at his team at work. His behavior was almost manic, but he wasn't bipolar. And anytime he stopped drinking coffee, he'd completely crash.

After we ran an adrenal test, his symptoms suddenly made sense: His cortisol was through the roof in the morning and didn't drop all day. This is what is called phase 1 adrenal fatigue. He didn't have a disease, but his brain was pushing his adrenals to pump out all this cortisol and epinephrine just to keep him going. To help lower his cortisol levels, I suggested he stop drinking coffee, which caused him to crash for a few days, but it had to be done in order to stabilize his energy levels and lower stress on his system. He also needed to start sleeping eight hours per night, meditating, and eating three meals a day instead of drinking ten cups of coffee and having dinner only. These simple things got his cortisol—and his behavior—back in line.

Some of my patients have the opposite problem: Their cortisol levels are too low, morning, noon, and night. These are my patients who can't get out of bed in the morning and just feel exhausted all day, every day. They've pushed their bodies to the brink, either with too much stress, too little sleep, or both, and their adrenals have essentially given up, incapable of mounting a normal up-and-down cortisol response. I see this happen often with moms, especially after they have a second or third child. For example, one young mother came to see me ten months after delivering baby #2, showing up in my office pale, thin, and exhausted. She almost looked as though she was made of paper—I felt like if a strong breeze came through the office window, it might cause her to lose her balance. Even standing up seemed like effort. She thought she might be depressed and told me she wanted to see a psychiatrist.

Some of her exhaustion was understandable, of course: She was working full-time with two young kids at home, and although her youngest had started to sleep through the night, she still wasn't getting a full night's rest. And she was still trying to go to the gym and push on with life, without, as she told me, much support from her partner. But all the stress of her life didn't account for her extreme exhaustion and depression.

When we tested her adrenals, I wasn't necessarily surprised to see that her cortisol had flatlined—it was literally a flat line instead of a curve. Her body could still make cortisol in the event of an emergency, giving her energy if, for example, she suddenly discovered that her newborn was choking or her older son had wandered off. But since she'd been stressed 24-7 for so long, her glands had simply stopped making the hormone on a healthy basis.

Helping her heal was more challenging, because her body needed a number of things, including deep rest; more water, omega-3 fats, fiber, and protein; and a reset of her stress response. We achieved this over time by helping her wean the baby so she was able to get a full night's sleep on a more regular basis, and could start going to bed earlier instead of staying up for an eleven o'clock feed. She started taking a combination of targeted herbal supplements that can aid in rebalancing what's known as the hypothalamus-pituitary-adrenal (HPA) axis, which helps regulate the body's stress response and energy levels. She even took a one-week doctor-prescribed beach vacation alone, the focus of which was to get sleep, sea, and sun, realizing that if she didn't ask her partner for support while she took a short break, it might break their marriage. This process took three to four months, which may sound like a long time, but as I told her: "You didn't get here in a week, so we can't undo this in a week." But eventually we were able to get her energy, stamina, and cortisol curve back into healthy levels.

Sex Hormones

If this is the section you've been waiting for, you may be surprised when I tell you that medical testing for sex hormones isn't prescribed as often as most people assume it would or should be. You'd think every doctor would always test for estrogen and testosterone, given their fundamental importance to our overall health. But unless you've had fertility or libido issues or asked your doctor explicitly, I doubt you've had your estrogen, testosterone, or progesterone levels checked recently.

One reason why no one is regularly screening for sex hormones, not even ob-gyns, is training. In med school, we learn that estrogen and testosterone are relatively frivolous compared to "real" health concerns. We're also not taught why someone's sex hormones may be abnormal in the first place, or what to do treat an imbalance other than replacing the hormones with synthetic medications like birth control pills. Even administering testosterone to men with low levels or hormone-replacement therapy (HRT) to women in menopause isn't really covered in med school, because it's considered "elective"—not necessary to basic health. And when synthetic hormones are used, they often don't fix the problem; they just mask whatever is really going on.

The reason I test my patients for sex hormonal imbalances is that they can be causing or worsening a mood disorder, or contributing to symptoms like fatigue, depression, low energy, sleep difficulties, and brain fog. Imbalances can also cause a host of physical problems, like weight gain, irregular periods, low libido, abnormal hair growth, and breast tissue growth in men. Sex hormones also don't work in a vacuum: They perform in partnership with your adrenal and thyroid hormones, which is why I think it's important to look at all three together to understand your entire hormonal operation.

Sex hormone testing is also important beyond the level of "elective" for women in menopause or nearing menopause. At Parsley, we test a woman's estrogen, progesterone, and testosterone to identify where she is in her cycle in her late forties and fifties. This way, we can try to mitigate menopause-related symptoms like poor sleep, weight gain, and depression before these symptoms get worse or require HRT.

No matter what age you are or what kind of imbalance you might have, you may not need or want a synthetic hormone, which can cause side effects worse than the symptoms of an imbalance. I treat a lot of hormonal imbalances with potent herbal supplements, stress management, and nutritional changes. But it's important to remember that hormonal imbalances do need to be treated in order to feel your best, so the first step is having the testing done.

Genetic Testing

While many people believe their genes determine their health, only 10 percent of our medical outcomes stem from our genes—the other 90 percent are the result of our environment and how we eat, move, and live. That's why in medical school we have the saying "Genetics load the gun, but environment pulls the trigger."

Still, that 10 percent is really important, especially if it's keeping you stuck in a flyover pattern of feeling tired, depressed, foggy, anxious, or unhappy. Here's where genetic testing comes in: It can be a huge hack to unlock why you feel the way you do and help get you to a better place, mentally and emotionally. At Parsley, we don't use complicated, costly tests, but rather relatively inexpensive, easy-to-access screenings like 23andMe and Ancestry.com to help patients in two major ways.

The first way is that we can take information provided by direct-to-consumer DNA tests or medical tests doctors can order, like Genomind, to help figure out if someone is taking the best antidepressant for their genetic makeup. By combining raw DNA information with a second online analytics tool that pinpoints certain genetic variants and how they might be affecting your health, we can determine how a person makes and breaks down certain neurotransmitters, like serotonin, norepinephrine, and dopamine. Since different antidepressants work by balancing these chemicals in different ways, we can then use this information to tailor-fit the right drug to a patient's unique metabolism. This can be a game-changer. Many times when I find patients can benefit from an antidepressant, they've been prescribed the wrong one because their psychiatrist hasn't used genetics to personalize their prescription.

The second way we use genetics to improve mental health at Parsley is by using the same information—how your body makes and breaks down neurotransmitters—to identify whether you may have a genetic variant that's affecting your mood in the first place. The most common one we see at Parsley involves the gene MTHFR, which may sound like a curse word, but it's actually a super-common genetic variant that can worsen depression or anxiety.

The MTHFR gene codes for an enzyme that converts the B vitamins folate and B_{12} into more usable forms known as methyl-folate and methyl-B_{12}, respectively, both which the body uses as essential building blocks for serotonin, norepinephrine, and dopamine. But if you inherited a variant of the MTHFR gene from either or both your parents, your body can't convert these Bs into their usable forms as quickly, disrupting your gut and your brain's ability to manufacture mood-stabilizing neurotransmitters. In addition, slow folate conversion can lead to a buildup of the amino acid homocysteine in your blood, which can trigger or worsen depression, anxiety, and chronic fatigue, as well as increase your risk factors for heart disease.

MTHFR gene variants are common: According to the CDC, more people have a variant than don't. I myself have a type of MTHFR variant, and for years, I had no idea that it was helping to fuel my anxiety, until I took a genetic test. Now I know that when I take methylated B_{12} and methylated folate in my multivitamin—which is how we treat MTHFR variants—I'm far more in control of my mood. These methylated B vitamins, which are more bioavailable than regular B vitamins, help the body clear excess homocysteine, help you build neurotransmitters, and limit the symptoms associated with MTHFR variants. We'll talk more about methylated Bs on page 199.

With genetic testing, I also learned that I have what's known as the "worrier" variant of something called the COMT gene, which helps code for certain enzymes in the brain. If you have the worrier variant like me, your brain is slow to get rid of excess dopamine, meaning more of the neurotransmitter remains active in your brain for a longer time. This is great for executive function and decision-making, but it's bad for worriers like me, since it can keep the brain on high alert. The opposite of the worrier variant is the "warrior" version, which means your brain processes dopamine quickly, which helps you stay calm under pressure but oftentimes triggers slower decision-making and poor concentration. Similar to MTHFR, specific supplementation can help support or even hack these gene variants.

Having a variant like MTHFR or COMT doesn't mean you have a disease, but it may mean you can benefit from taking certain supplements or adopting specific self-care routines, especially if a variant is causing you to feel anxious, bummed out, or burned out. For me, methylated Bs have made all the difference in my mood, and I'm not alone. At Parsley, we sell a prenatal vitamin that includes methylated Bs, and I can't tell you how many moms-to-be have told me the supplement overhauled their baseline outlook on life. The only problem: Methylated Bs aren't found in most multivitamins or prenatal supplements, even though they should be, in my opinion.

If I can prescribe a patient a B vitamin that works like an antidepressant, that's a huge win for everyone. And while methylated Bs won't magically cure either genetic variant condition or be enough to avoid medication on their own, they can significantly improve how some of us feel.

Beyond Basic Blood Sugar Testing

Blood sugar is usually overlooked as a marker for our mood and mental health. But think about it for a moment: If you're consuming massive amounts of sugar all day, as most Americans do, it's not going to end well for your brain or mental and emotional stability, for many of the reasons we've already discussed in previous chapters. In short, high blood sugar and insulin-resistance issues keep your mood strapped into an emotional roller coaster and can lead to brain inflammation and microbiome imbalances, both of which can cause or worsen depression, anxiety, brain fog, ADHD, and chronic fatigue.

Blood sugar is also a bit of a chicken-egg dilemma when it comes to your mental and emotional health. If you're eating a lot of sugar, as most people are, it can cause you to feel anxious, sad, foggy, or irritable. But if you already feel anxious, sad, foggy, or irritable, as many people do, you may crave sugar as a means of self-soothing, since sugar spikes dopamine in the brain to hit us with a temporary feel-good effect. In part for this reason, I've never seen a single patient who can't benefit from in-depth blood sugar testing and better blood sugar regulation.

You would think regular and comprehensive blood sugar testing would be automatic, given that two-thirds of all Americans are overweight or obese, one-third have diabetes or prediabetes, and another third have metabolic syndrome—a dangerous disorder that increases the risk of heart disease, diabetes, depression, anxiety, and other physical and mental health problems. But over and over again, I see new patients in their thirties, forties, and fifties who've never had their blood sugar thoroughly or consistently checked and who have metabolic syndrome, prediabetes, or full-fledged diabetes.

Basic blood work ordered by most primary care clinics will usually include a test for hemoglobin A1C, which can indicate elevated blood sugar levels. But few people actually have or regularly see a primary care doctor, and if they do, that physician may not be ordering basic blood work often enough, as blood sugar levels can change every three months.

Finally, A1C doesn't tell the whole story of someone's blood sugar—in fact, it's pretty limited. I also test for fasting insulin and fasting glucose at least once if not

80

twice a year, both of which can reveal a blood sugar issue long before an A1C test will.

Autoimmune Testing

People think of the immune system as their friend—and generally, it is. When you suffer a sinus infection or break a bone, your immune system goes into attack mode, fighting off the bad stuff and cleaning up inflammation to send you on your healthy and happy way.

But the way we live today has turned many of our immune systems from a friend to a foe. High sugar consumption, frequent antibiotic use, and exposure to chemicals and additives in our food supply have collectively caused many of our immune systems to become confused. The result for 50 million Americans is an autoimmune disorder, which occurs when the immune system turns its firepower on itself and begins attacking the body, even the healthy parts.

While autoimmune disorders like Crohn's disease, psoriasis, rheumatoid arthritis, and Hashimoto's thyroiditis are common, especially among women (who account for 80 percent of all autoimmune condition diagnoses), they get missed all the time. People with autoimmune diseases will see an average of six doctors over four years before getting a proper diagnosis. In the meantime, they're dealing with many of the hallmark symptoms of autoimmune conditions, including fatigue, weight gain, brain fog, headaches, irritability, depression, joint pain, nerve damage, and/or acne. And if you do discover you have an autoimmune disorder, you have a 25 percent chance of developing a second one in your lifetime. Here's the real kicker: Testing for most autoimmune disorders is relatively easy, requiring only a simple blood draw. For all new Parsley patients, I run an ANA test, or antinuclear antibody test, which can show whether your immune system cells are attacking the nuclei of your healthy cells. With the same blood test, I can also check for certain inflammatory markers, including erythrocyte sedimentation rate (ESR) and high-sensitivity C-reactive protein (hsCRP), both of which can indicate systemic inflammation as the result of an autoimmune disorder. And Parsley's standard thyroid panel includes a test for TPO antibodies, which screens for Hashimoto's thyroiditis.

If a patient's blood work shows high levels of inflammation, I might also test to see if he or she has a food sensitivity, intolerance, or allergy that's triggering that inflammation. But I don't automatically check for food sensitivities and allergies on Day One unless I strongly suspect one. There are smarter ways to identify food issues, which we'll detail in Chapter Six.

Autoimmune testing can have a profound effect on your physical, mental, and emotional health. I still remember the first time I discovered an autoimmune condition in a patient—a good friend who came to see me soon after I started practicing. My friend had been struggling with depression for years, along with irritability and fatigue, and nothing was adding up. When I checked his TSH levels—the basic test for thyroid function—everything was normal, but when we ran tests for ANA and Hashimoto's antibodies, it was like someone had suddenly switched on a light: He clearly had the condition.

Soon after we started treating his Hashimoto's, my friend's life changed: His irritability and fatigue went away, and we were slowly able to wean him off the antidepressant Zoloft, which he had taken for some time despite no significant improvements in his mood. This was another lightbulb moment for me: If the underlying cause of depression or anxiety is due to too much inflammation and not a serotonin issue, then serotonin-targeting antidepressants probably won't help that much! Years later, I still remember my friend's story because it changed my entire perception of what I thought I knew and what I'd been taught in school. Today, at Parsley, we've been able to change so many other lives in similar ways by testing for and treating autoimmune diseases.

Stage Two Immunity Testing

If a patient is struggling with many of the hallmark signs of an autoimmune disease—fatigue, depression, joint pain, etc.—but doesn't have elevated antibody or inflammatory markers, I'll consider doing next-step testing for three illnesses that can cause an autoimmune or autoimmune-like reaction: Lyme disease, Epstein-Barr virus, and the illness that comes from toxic mold exposure. These infections are less common than autoimmune disorders but still all too real for those who suffer with them. They're also difficult to diagnose and are usually poorly understood and often overlooked by conventional doctors.

Lyme disease isn't an autoimmune condition in itself, but it can trigger an autoimmune reaction called post-treatment Lyme disease syndrome (PTLDS) in some people. PTLDS causes many of the same symptoms of an autoimmune disorder, including chronic fatigue, brain fog, anxiety, depression, and headaches. The blood test we use to identify Lyme disease is rudimentary at best, but I'll still administer it to patients if I suspect they may have been infected.

Similar to Lyme, Epstein-Barr virus (EBV) can create an autoimmune reaction in some people. The virus, part of the herpes family, infects 90 percent of all adults, most of whom don't experience health issues as a result. But a small percentage of people develop something called post-EBV inflammatory syndrome that's very similar to PTLDS, causing the immune system to attack healthy cells. Post-EBV syndrome can be detected through a blood test that screens for EBV antibodies.

Toxic mold illness, also referred to as a biotoxin illness, occurs when someone is exposed to too much mold and develops an autoimmune reaction, with similar symptoms to an autoimmune disorder, including brain fog, fatigue, anxiety, and depression. If I suspect toxic mold illness, I'll order both blood and urine tests to try to figure out whether mold is being excreted from the kidneys or is causing systemic immune disruption.

One of the best emails I've received was a note a couple of years ago from Dr. Rita Charon, one of the top professors at Columbia Medical School. She wrote that one of her patient's children had been sick with symptoms that suggested a kidney issue but that no one could figure it out. The child came to see a pediatrician at Parsley, who ran our standard panel of diagnostic testing to try to identify what might be wrong with the boy. When the initial screens came up negative, we took it one step further and ran stage-two tests for immunity, only to find that the boy had a bad case of toxic mold illness. Our pediatrician recommended the child's home be thoroughly and naturally cleaned (I emphasize *naturally* because toxic household cleaners carry their own set of health problems) and treated the boy to help remove biotoxins from his body. Within a couple of months, the child's health had been fully restored. While I didn't personally treat the boy, Dr. Charon wrote to congratulate me on operating a practice that was willing to think outside the box in medicine. My heart basically exploded with joy.

The story illustrates what we see happen all the time: People, even those with access to some of the best medical care in the world, aren't getting the right diagnoses because they're not getting the right diagnostic tests. Identifying a condition like toxic mold illness takes investigative work and nontraditional thinking, which most conventional doctors don't have the time, bandwidth, or training for.

Nutrient Deficiency Testing

Many people think nutrient deficiencies happen primarily in developing countries or only to the very old or infirm. After all, food in the United States is everywhere, and much of it is fortified with extra nutrients.

But the truth is, we live in a calorie-dense, nutrient-poor country. Most Americans are overfed but undernourished. That's because our standard American diet of ultrarefined, ultra-processed foods is low in vitamins, minerals, healthy fats, fiber, antioxidants, and phytonutrients—chemicals produced by plants that help the body fight disease—all of which are essential to optimal physical, mental, and emotional function. For this reason, as many as nine out of every ten Americans are deficient in at least one essential nutrient, or a vitamin, mineral, or other food-based chemical cofactor the body needs for optimal physical function. If you take into account those nutrients that aren't considered essential by the FDA, including marine omega-3 fats, antioxidants, and phytonutrients, our collective nutrient deficiency is much higher.

Even if you're eating fatty fish and green vegetables around the clock and see that as proof positive you're getting all the nutrients you need, that doesn't necessarily mean your body is absorbing or even using those nutrients. I see plenty of patients with health conditions that cause malabsorption, including leaky gut syndrome; irritable bowel syndrome; hypothyroidism; Crohn's disease; yeast or bacterial overgrowth; food sensitivities, intolerances, or allergies; or certain genetic variants, some of which we already discussed (see pages 78–79). Malabsorption can't usually be solved with supplements either, since the body has a more difficult time absorbing or using a nutrient from a pill than it does a natural food source.

Drinking too much alcohol or caffeine or being stressed out all the time can limit nutrient absorption, which is also true of many common medications like birth control pills, antacids, antidepressants, ADHD drugs, and antianxiety pills. What's more, industrially farmed vegetables, fruits, grains, and other crops now contain fewer nutrients than they did decades ago, due to soil depletion and rising levels of carbon dioxide (which make plants grow bigger, not more nutritious). That means we're all eating fewer naturally occurring nutrients than our parents and grandparents did. And then there's the problem with the toxins in our food, air, water, household cleaners, personal-care products, and general environment, all of which can interfere with the body's ability to absorb vitamins, minerals, and other key nutrients.

Add up all these reasons, and it may not be surprising to learn that you might absorb only 10 percent of a nutrient from any given food. So even if you diet is amazing—and I'm guessing it may not be—you still have a good chance of having a nutrient deficiency.

At Parsley I see a lot of people who aren't getting the nutrition they need to feel happy, calm, and focused, let alone to have proper physical function and long-term health. The most common deficiencies we see in the practice are in B vitamins, particularly B_{12} and folate, a lack of which can cause exhaustion, depression, anxiety, sleep problems, and a host of other mental issues. We also have a lot of patients who are low in the kind of nutrients that are essential for good thyroid function, including selenium, zinc, iodine, iron, and vitamin D. Vitamin D deficiency is extremely common, with some reports suggesting that 94 percent of all Americans fall below the estimated average requirement. In addition to thyroid issues, low vitamin D levels can also cause poor immune function and muscle pain, along with fatigue and depression.

Many patients, particularly women, are iron deficient, but it goes undetected because doctors are looking at blood count, which is a late sign you're iron deficient, instead of proactively testing for ferritin. Ferritin is how we measure iron stores, which is an early indicator of whether you're low on iron. Low ferritin levels can produce the same issues as iron-deficiency anemia, including fatigue, but most doctors, even if they suspect anemia, don't test a patient's ferritin.

I see women, many who are mothers, who literally have a hard time climbing the stairs off the subway to make it to our New York City office not because they're out of shape but because they're so tired from low iron stores. I see the same mom-exhaustion memes all over social media—*Friend: "You look tired." Mom: "I have kids. I'm pretty sure that's just my face now."*—but for many, they're not exhausted simply because their toddler won't sleep a full eight hours but because they literally don't have the reserve iron to make enough red blood cells.

With new patients, I also like to order an omega-3 index, which measures levels of the two marine omega-3 fatty acids, eicosapentaenoic acid (EPA) and docosahexaenoic acid (DHA). Ninety-five percent of all Americans—yes, that's basically *all* of us—don't get enough EPA and DHA, which are found primarily in seafood, and in much lesser amounts in seaweed, algae (spirulina), chicken, and eggs. Our ubiquitous lack of marine omega-3s is a problem, since EPA and DHA are essential not only to immune function but also to brain function: Sixty percent of the brain is made up of fat, a large part of which should be omega-3 fat for optimal function. Without enough EPA and DHA, your brain can't operate optimally, and your risk of cognitive decline and mood disorders like depression shoots up. Don't get me wrong: Americans are definitely eating enough fat—we're just not eating the right kind. For example, we're getting plenty of omega-6 fats, found mostly in refined vegetable oils and processed, packaged foods. Today, our ratio of omega-6 to omega-3 fats is up to 20:1 on average. To put that number into perspective, your omega-6 to omega-3 ratio should be 4:1 or lower for optimal cellular and immune health. Having too much omega-6 drives up brain inflammation and the risk of depression, anxiety, and other mental health issues, in addition to physical problems.

If you're dealing with severe depression or anxiety, a nutrient deficiency may not be causing the issue, but it's certainly not helping you address it. What I tell my patients is that nutrient deficiencies can worsen other conditions or generally contribute to a "lack of resilience," or a reduced ability to deal with whatever life throws your way. Identifying and correcting these deficiencies, no matter how major or minor they might be, basically helps ensure that your body is playing with a full deck of cards, ready to throw down whatever nutrient it needs in order to counter life's inevitable physiological and psychological stressors.

Despite the fact most people aren't playing with a full nutritional deck, testing for nutrients is hardly standard care. In med school, we're taught that nutrient deficiencies are severe afflictions that only people like sailors get after being out at sea for months, developing scurvy because they didn't have access to fresh fruits and vegetables with vitamin C. I don't know about my colleagues, but I have yet to see a sailor or anyone else with scurvy walk into my office, even though there were several questions about the condition on my board exams.

What I see far more often than sailors with scurvy is patients like Beth, a tall, sweet woman in her mid-fifties who came to see me for chronic fatigue. Her exhaustion had become so severe that she was barely able to work as a third-grade teacher anymore. This frightened her: She had become a teacher at an elementary school because she loved it and thought it would be a great job for life— something that would take her through retirement. But while she still loved her kids, suddenly she was feeling "over it" and was actually starting to consider quitting to take time off.

I ordered all the diagnostic tests for Beth that I do for all my new patients, and what we discovered was that not only did she have two copies of the variant of the MTHFR gene, she was also extremely low in ferritin, which no doctor had tested for despite some obvious signs of anemia. Beth also had a very poor omega-3 fatty acid score, which was interfering with her ability to manage inflammation.

I immediately started Beth on liquid iron—formulated as ferrous bisglycinate, which is the form the body can best absorb—mixed with vitamin C, which increases absorption further. She also started taking my favorite methylated B vitamins for her MTHFR variants, as well as an omega-3 supplement with potent levels of EPA and DHA. Within about two months, Beth's exhaustion had receded, and she slowly began to emerge from her fog, returning to work with the same enthusiasm and energy she had felt when she started more than twenty years ago.

The Answers Are in the Gut: Digestive Health Testing

The gut: What is even going on in there? For most of us, our gastrointestinal tract is a mystery—and one we'd rather not think about too hard. Instead, we expect it to quietly digest our food, praying it doesn't bother us otherwise. The problem, though, is that our gut is the root of our health and often the real cause behind what's going on in our bodies and brains. Thankfully, new developments in testing over the past few years have made it easier to discover what's really happening inside our GI tract.

To be clear, the following digestive-health tests are not standard first-step screening practices for new patients at Parsley. But we run them all the time as second-step testing because they're often a huge unlock for people's mental health, for three reasons: (1) digestive health issues can and do often cause mood disorders, (2) more and more people are suffering from the gut issues that lead to mood problems, and (3) few doctors test for or even know about the digestive-health issues that can cause mood disorders.

The two digestive-health tests that I most frequently order are a hydrogen-methane breath test and a three-day stool test. We order these tests primarily for patients who have persistent digestive issues alongside brain fog—the presence of both is a good indicator someone has something wrong in their gut microbiome.

I've used the term *microbiome* already, and you may already be familiar with the concept: The body's universe of trillions of microorganisms inside the gut has certainly been in the spotlight recently, as doctors have uncovered more about all the ways in which our microbiome affects our health. One reason the microbiome is so influential is because your body and its DNA are more microbial than human—only 43 percent of you is made up of human cells and human genes. This means what happens in your microorganism community has a profound impact on your physiological and psychological health.

When it comes to mood, the microbiome influences a lot. Ninety-five percent of the body's serotonin, or feel-good hormone, is produced in the gut, along with other neurotransmitters, like dopamine, GABA, and norepinephrine, all which are critical to mood regulation. Perhaps more significantly, your microbiome is connected directly to your brain via a two-way highway known as the gut-brain axis: Whenever something happens inside your gut, it directly affects your brain and vice versa.

The gut-brain axis is not a minor road but a major interstate freeway. Research shows that when people change the composition of their microbiome by consuming food, alcohol, supplements, medication, and/or toxins, the brain responds in kind, triggering different behaviors or moods depending on what you ingested. For example, scientists have found that when women eat more yogurt with probiotics, or healthy bacteria, they respond more calmly to emotional tasks after just four weeks, according to brain imaging. With 70 percent to 80 percent of all our immune cells in our microbiome, our gut also helps control inflammation, including in the brain. In short, an unhealthy gut can lead to an inflamed brain, increasing the risk of depression, irritability, sadness, anxiety, brain fog, ADHD, and general malaise.

How do you know if you have an unhealthy gut? In today's world, microbiome imbalances are common, thanks to what we eat (sugar, carbs, unhealthy fat, not enough fiber, not enough micronutrients), what we drink (alcohol, caffeine, more sugar), how we move (we don't), the medications we take (antibiotics, antidepressants, acid blockers, painkillers, laxatives), the toxins we're exposed to in our environment, our lack of sleep, our addiction to screens, and even our elevated stress levels. Many common health conditions can also impact your microbiome, including having food sensitivities, autoimmune disorders, high blood sugar, or being overweight or obese.

For people with bloating, burping, acid reflux, easily feeling full after light meals, and intermittent constipation and diarrhea, we take a look at the upper digestive tract, otherwise known as the small intestine. In these patients, we run something called a hydrogen/methane breath test. The test, which requires a patient to blow into a bag after drinking a sugar solution, can identify whether you have small intestinal bacterial overgrowth (SIBO), which happens when bad bacteria take over your small intestine and cause symptoms like bloating, gas, brain fog, and even rosacea. If you have SIBO, the bacteria in the small intestine devour the sugar solution and produce gases, which are picked up by the breath test. The test can also tell us which types of bacteria may exist in your gut at what levels, allowing us to treat your SIBO even more effectively.

For people with irritable bowel symptoms like bloating, diarrhea, constipation, bleeding, and/or gas, we take a look at their lower digestive tract, or colon, by using a three-day stool test. As fun as this sounds, it's actually easy to do at home, and the results can be highly valuable. The test helps identify the presence of inflammation, parasites, yeast overgrowth, poor digestive function, or too few helpful bacteria, all of which can disrupt your mental health. And while the test may sound disgusting, it's really clean: We give patients small containers, and all you have to do is take a teeny-tiny sample of your poo each day.

We'll talk more about how to treat gut issues throughout the book, but if you have SIBO, a yeast overgrowth, gut inflammation, or another digestive-health issue interfering with your mood or mental health, you don't have to overhaul your life in order to fix the problem. Oftentimes, we can treat digestive-health issues with potent herbal supplements, prescription medication, and/or a gut-healing protocol.

Remember my patient Alyssa, who was dealing with severe bloating, gas, brain fog, and ADHD when she first came to see me several years ago (page 15)? She's a prime example of how you can hack your mental health using these tests. When we met, the thirty-four-year-old had been on migraine medication and the ADHD drug Adderall for years, but still had headaches and brain fog all the time. From her health biography, I knew she had been on rounds of antibiotics for sinus infections for years and that she ate too much sugar. From her symptom index, I could see that her brain fog and digestive issues traveled together. This made her an ideal candidate for a breath test, which showed us she had SIBO. Once we started treating it, her indigestion, brain fog, and headaches all went away, and we were able to get her off the prescription meds. This was a huge win: Alyssa gained her life back in a matter of months, and felt ready to try to have the baby she'd always wanted.

Your Diagnostic Testing Cheat Sheet

You've just learned about a lot of different diagnostic tests, and if you're feeling a little overwhelmed right now, I don't blame you. But the onus of testing isn't on you: You will need to have a doctor to help steer your through your journey to better health. Most tests in this chapter are ones that primary care doctors should understand or be able to reference on the platforms that we doctors use to ensure we stay on top of the latest research. While you may have to ask your primary care doctor to order these tests, remember: It's your life, your health, your body, your mind, and your mood that will affect you every day, not theirs. If you have access to a functional or integrative doctor who's trained in more proactive testing, you may get more insight (we'll discuss this further in Chapter Ten). But bottom line: Testing is a critical step in your journey to have a State Change and overhaul your health and how you feel.

To make it easier for you to have the right conversation with your doctor, here are the tests to ask him or her for:

- Thyroid
  Thyroid-stimulating hormone (TSH)
  Free T4
  Free T3
  Anti-TPO
  Antithyroglobulin
- Adrenal
  - five-point cortisol test via urine or saliva
- Sex Hormones
  Estrogen as Estradiol, Estriol, and Estrone
  Progesterone
  Testosterone
- Genetic Testing
  MTHFR variant
  COMT variant
  Assessment for most effective antidepressant class
- Blood Sugar
  Hemoglobin A1C
  Fasting insulin
  Fasting glucose
- Autoimmune Testing
  Antinuclear antibody test (ANA)

Erythrocyte sedimentation rate (ESR)

High-sensitivity C-reactive protein (hsCRP)

- Stage Two Immune

Lyme disease test

Epstein-Barr virus test

Toxic mold illness using blood and urine tests

- Nutrient Basis

Vitamin B_{12}

Folate

Vitamin D_3

Magnesium

Selenium

Iodine

Zinc

Hematocrit, hemoglobin, and ferritin stores (iron)

Omega-3 index

Ferritin

- Digestive Health

Hydrogen/methane breath test

Three-day stool test (e.g., GI Effects from Genova Diagnostics)

I want to reiterate what I said at the beginning of this chapter: With just a few exceptions, most of these tests are simple to do, easy for your doctor to order, covered by insurance, and require only one trip to the lab for a blood draw. I also want to emphasize that you have the right to ask for every single test listed here. Asking your doctor for a diagnostic screening doesn't make you high-maintenance or obnoxious: It makes you a person who cares about your health and is proactive and passionate about living a healthier, happier life. In my opinion, that's the best kind of patient to be. What's more, these tests can help your doctor better treat you: If you're suffering from a thyroid disorder, blood sugar imbalance, digestive-health issue, or any other manageable condition, identifying it now will save you and your doctor time, effort, and potential angst down the road.

I'm not saying that getting these tests won't take time, money, and effort—it will. But this is one of the most important things you can do to set your body, mind, and mood up for success. Testing will allow you to understand what's driving your symptoms, connect the dots between what's happening in your body and what's happening in your mind, and get ahead of possible problems before they get serious. Remember, you didn't get here in a day, and it will take more than a day to resolve your mental health issues. And if you've been suffering from brain fog, fatigue, anxiety, depression, irritability, or any other mood disorder, the time and effort it takes to get these tests are just a drop in the bucket compared to living the rest of your life with sadness, worry, anger, fogginess, insomnia, or fuzziness. These tests can change your life—I've seen it with many of my patients—and help you get to a whole new level of health and happiness. Ultimately, they're a critical step to take toward your first State Change.

CHAPTER FIVE

Move the Energy

N ot speaking to another human being for ten days straight is really, really hard. Not moving is even harder.

Rewind twelve years to an open-air temple in the middle of the jungle two hours north of Bangkok, and that's exactly what I was doing: not speaking and not moving. And that's how I learned something about exercise that has influenced how I treat my patients with mental health issues ever since. It's why I won't prescribe antidepressants to any patient who doesn't move his or her body in a meaningful way on a near-daily basis and why I personally try to be active as much as I can be—not just because I want to look good in a bathing suit but because I want to stay sane and feel good in my mind.

Let me explain. And let me start in Thailand.

I didn't mean to go to Thailand. The summer after my first year in medical school at Columbia, I volunteered to do work in Nepal, helping an international nonprofit screen women for cervical cancer. Nepal is known as the gateway to the Himalayas. It's also a soul seeker's destination, popular with people looking for spiritual enlightenment, with its thousands of Buddhist stupas and temples dotted across the countryside like white and gold mushrooms, many adorned with flickering butter lamps, spinning temple bells, and rainbows of fluttering prayer flags. It's a beautiful country, but one where technology and healthcare standards, particularly for women, are stuck in the last century.

I was in Nepal to help a public health group funded by the US Agency for International Development (USAID) improve women's health. My work focused on a research project that took me across the country assessing standards of gynecological care. I wasn't there to be enlightened or for any particular spiritual purpose, but I was surrounded by those who were. From the European backpacker kids, international aid workers, and aspiring mountaineers whom I met while drinking chai tea in Kathmandu, I kept hearing about something called Vipassana, a ten-day silent meditation retreat that many credited with transforming their lives. As the summer wore on and I met more and more people who told me how incredible the retreat was, I decided that I had to try it. An hour in a fluorescent-lit internet café later, I found a Vipassana center in Thailand with spots available at the end of August, and I signed up, postponing my flights back to the US by two weeks despite my parents' protests. When else would I ever have the opportunity to do something like this again?

Weeks later, I boarded a plane from Kathmandu to Bangkok. After exploring the city for a few days, I took a hot, jumpy bus to the Vipassana center, carved out of the jungle several hundred miles north of the capital. The center was modest, with one large, open main temple, where women were instructed to sit on one side and men on the other. This is where we would sit and meditate for ten hours every day, without speaking, reading, writing, or making eye contact with one another. The only noises were the birds outside the temple screens and the sound of instructions piped through loudspeakers in both Thai and English on how to perform each day's meditation.

Sitting, meditating, and abstaining from all social interaction for ten days in a row is absolutely one of the hardest things I've ever done. When you first arrive at the center, you hand over your phone, camera, books, and any reading or writing materials, meaning you have no distractions. I slept in a room the size of a small cell and shared showers and a bathroom with birds, lizards, and others from the retreat. The temple gong woke us up each day at 4:30 in the morning for the first meditation session, and we took breaks only for breakfast, lunch, and late-afternoon tea—there was no dinner.

The only exception to this eat-sleep-meditate cycle was, at the end of each day, the instructors played a thirty-minute video narrated by Satya Narayan Goenka, the Indian teacher who founded Vipassana, who explained the practice's philosophy and why we were doing what we were doing. This is where I first heard something about human biology that would change my perception of patient care forever:

Emotions don't just live in the head:
They also live in the body.

As Goenka explained, every time you think a thought or feel an emotion, it triggers a cascade of hormones, neurotransmitters, and other chemicals in the body and brain. If you think the same thoughts or feel the same emotions over and over again, this biochemical cascade keeps happening, eventually altering the activity and structure of the cells in both your body and brain. Depending on what you feel, whether positive or negative, this cascade and the consequent cellular changes are either helpful or harmful to your overall physical and mental health. The consequences of repetitive thought patterns, particularly negative ones, are physical changes in your body—in your muscles, bones, nerves, and organs—that can ultimately result in illness. Goenka founded Vipassana after years of migraines that not even the top doctors in Asia could help fix. He ultimately found that a practice of releasing stored emotions and thoughts from the tissues of the body through his particular style of meditation was the only thing that worked. He then created Vipassana to bring it to the world.

The concept resonated with me, but early in my medical training, I wasn't sure if this was just woo-woo talk or a fringe spiritual practice from the other side of the planet. In the years after the retreat, I learned that conventional science also recognizes the fact that emotions create a biochemical cascade, triggering hormones like cortisol (the body's stress hormone), neurotransmitters, and neuropeptides (small proteins released by brain cells) in the body and brain. When the body produces enough of the same chemicals over and over again, our cells adapt and change to better handle this continual chemical onslaught. What Goenka had discovered through his meditation practice, Western science had also confirmed in the lab.

The practice of Vipassana didn't just teach me that emotions live in my body; it also showed me, paradoxically through the act of sitting all day for eleven-plus hours, that exercise is the primary way through which we process our emotions on a daily basis, and is especially critical if your daily life doesn't include hours upon hours of focused meditation. All I needed was a ten-day experience that deprived me of almost all movement to show me exactly why.

The thing is, sitting completely still for eleven hours a day without moving an arm or even twitching a toe isn't easy—it's actually really, really physically painful. Different body parts start to fall asleep, and all the muscles you need to use to hold yourself erect and stationary start to cramp. During the retreat, pain roved through my body like a silent spider. I'd feel a sharp ache in my butt that would then migrate to my lower back, travel over my hip, move up my torso, and sit on my shoulder. I continually wanted to get up, walk around, and shake out my legs and arms, but that's exactly what you're not supposed to do in Vipassana: working through the pain using meditation instead of movement is a deliberate part of the process.

Thankfully, you're not left to your own devices to figure out how to overcome discomfort. During the retreat, the teachers guided us through a body scan meditation, in which you focus all your attention and awareness on the top of the head, then move through your body, concentrating on every individual part until you finish at the tips of your toes. Whenever you come across a tight or painful place, you focus on the pain until it moves or changes shape. The obstacle, as they say, is the way.

According to Goenka, as the pain moves or ebbs under your fully present observation, the practice allows you to release trapped emotions that live inside the body. This is one of the primary aims of Vipassana: Sit for hours on end and experience the pain and the past regrets, fears, and traumas that come along with it from a neutral perspective, then learn to release the pain, letting go of stuck emotions and old patterns of thought alongside it.

I was skeptical at first, but as I worked to release the pain through meditation, I could actually feel my body letting go of old feelings. Past memories flitted through my mind—everything from bad breakups to fights with friends and interactions I had had with my parents that I hadn't thought about for years. It felt as though I was continually releasing tiny traumas—not dismissing them as though nothing had happened but releasing the emotional energy I had chosen to store in my body on their behalf. As the retreat went on, I began to feel the same sense of lightness, calm, and contentment I had experienced over and over again through only one other activity: exercise.

That's when I connected the dots. At the time, I knew there was strong research showing that exercise benefits mental health, and I had certainly experienced these benefits myself through running or yoga. But I didn't realize until I was at Vipassana that our bodies are literally storage lockers for our emotions. When those emotions don't have an outlet, whether it's a mental outlet like meditation or a physical outlet like movement, they don't leave the body—they get trapped inside, causing biochemical disruptions that can wreak havoc on our physical, mental, and emotional health. Several years later, when I started seeing patients as a doctor, I began to see this over and over again: Those patients who didn't move their bodies in a meaningful way on a regular basis almost always came into my office with some kind of mood instability, coupled with physical issues.

In other words, your issues are in your tissues. And it's entirely possible for you to get your issues out of your tissues, even those that have existed inside your body for years, causing physical, mental, and emotional damage. Vipassana—or any type of meditation—is a powerful way to release negative emotions and end the harmful biochemical cascade these feelings can cause, but it's not the only way. In our modern Western lifestyles where taking an hour to meditate—let alone ten days—feels impossible, prolonged focused meditation is simply not an avenue most people use to manage their feelings. Physical movement is another way, and in my opinion, it's an absolutely necessary way to help detoxify and expel negative emotions and prevent that chemical buildup, which, over time, will destroy your physical and mental health. That's one big reason why exercise feels so good: It's not just because you're getting an endorphin rush or improved blood flow—you're actually processing out negative emotions and stopping a potentially harmful biochemical barrage. You're literally getting your issues out of your tissues.

This realization that I first made in Thailand corroborated what I had begun to understand while doing medical research at New York University. Before I went to medical school, I'd spent nearly a year studying how ADHD medications affected adult patients' brains as part of NYU's Mental Health and Addictive Disorders Research Program. The research required frequent interaction with patients in the trial, and over the course of the year, I got to know their daily habits very well. We spoke a lot about how they tried to manage their attention and energy imbalances outside of taking prescription drugs, and many of them had developed intense, highly personalized coping mechanisms. Some ate a ton of sugary foods to try to fix their mood problems, since sugar temporarily boosts dopamine, a neurotransmitter that improves mood, executive function, and focus. Others had crafted elaborate systems of daily checklists and reminders to help keep them on track so they could hold down a job or manage a family.

But out of the dozens of patients taking part in the trial, the people who self-managed their symptoms the best were those who exercised, many working out for over an hour per day because they had learned through experience that physical activity could boost their ability to focus and stabilize their energy for hours if not days afterward. These were the patients who were best able to hold down jobs, succeed in school, or manage households. While many of these hyper-exercisers still benefited from taking Adderall or similar medications as part of their regimen, they didn't need pills to make it through life.

If you've spent time with kids, you've likely witnessed this phenomenon firsthand: When children don't get to move around to get their willies out, they have a meltdown or temper tantrum. While most adults have learned how to control or suppress their emotions, the phenomenon is still there: When we don't move around to get our willies out, we have the adult version of a meltdown, allowing our negative emotions to fester and foment trouble inside us until we feel anxious, depressed, irritable, burned out, or cloudy and confused. This is a big reason why people who don't exercise are twice as likely to be depressed and 60 percent more likely to suffer anxiety, according to studies.

Bottom line: You can't sit and stew in your own emotional juices. You have to move your body in a meaningful way on a consistent basis over time. For this reason, exercise isn't a *nice-to-have* for mood stability and mental health: it's absolutely mandatory. Whether or not you care about getting fit, losing weight, or looking better in a bikini, you need to start working out and moving out old emotions before those emotions eat you alive.

The Three Big Ways Movement Improves Mood, Focus, and Energy

Knowing the science of why exercise is critical to mood can help you better understand why the practice isn't optional but integral to feeling good and having the kind of State Change that can transform your life.

1. Exercise is just as effective as antidepressants (if not more so), with additional perks and zero side effects.

Antidepressants might as well be in the water supply, that's how common they are in the US. Studies show that up to one in every six Americans takes at least one psychiatric drug, which includes medication like antidepressants and antianxiety pills. These estimates are likely higher in light of the COVID-19 pandemic, when prescriptions for antidepressants shot up by more than 18 percent and antianxiety prescriptions increased by more than 34 percent.

While it's wonderful that psychiatric drugs have become largely destigmatized in society and that people are getting the help they need, what's not so amazing is that their use—and in some instances, overuse—has distracted us from how everyday core actions can ease symptoms of depression and anxiety as successfully as drugs.

One of the most powerful everyday actions for optimal mood and mental health is regular exercise, which research has routinely shown is just as effective as prescription medication in treating depression. In fact, some studies show physical activity can treat some depression and anxiety more efficiently than drugs. In one trial, for example, 95 percent of psychiatric patients reported better mood after exercise. By comparison, a separate study found only 40 to 60 percent of patients noticed an improvement in depressive symptoms after taking prescription drugs for six to eight weeks.

Efficacy aside, there are reasons why exercise is a smart treatment choice for most people with mood problems: Unlike antidepressant and antianxiety drugs, exercise doesn't have negative side effects like weight gain, low libido, dizziness, sleepiness, and nausea. Quite the opposite: Being active can improve symptoms by stabilizing blood sugar, increasing metabolism, stimulating weight loss, adding lean muscle mass, boosting libido, sharpening cognitive function, enhancing sleep, and reducing disease risk, in addition to other benefits. All this in turn can increase feelings of confidence, self-esteem, and well-being. In other words, exercise accomplishes most of what people want for their bodies and brains.

I want to take the time here to stress that antidepressant medications can be critical, even lifesaving, for some people, no matter how much they exercise. But in my opinion, there are too many people who don't feel that good, mentally or emotionally, even though they've taken antidepressants for years. While drugs can help them climb out of the basement and onto the first floor so they can function in life with more stability—which is essential—these medications aren't helping them climb any higher. The only way to get to the next level is by moving on a regular, consistent basis. That's why I always make sure my patients are moving their bodies in meaningful ways on a daily basis before I prescribe psychiatric drugs, and emphasize that exercise doesn't go out the window once they start taking the drug. The meds are wonderful tools, but they'll never replace the methods in this book for creating a State Change.

2. Exercise is nature's best sleep aid.

One out of every three Americans doesn't get enough sleep, according to the CDC. In my practice, at least half of my patients don't sleep well, meaning they have trouble either falling asleep, staying asleep, or getting enough quality sleep. Remember, you can spend eight hours in bed every night but still not get enough deep sleep—one of the most important stages for the body and brain. A good indicator that you lack high-quality sleep is if you continually wake up feeling tired after seven or eight hours in bed.

While there's a pervasive sociocultural construct that we don't need sleep—people often brag that they don't sleep more than five hours a night, as though that's some sign of how successful or busy they are—chronic sleep deprivation is one of the worst things you can do for your mood. Just one night of inadequate sleep, for example, can drive anxiety levels up by a whopping 30 percent, to the point where researchers can detect significant changes in brain activity in imaging scans. Not getting enough shut-eye can also lead to feelings of stress, confusion, anger, irritability, loneliness, and sadness that, over time, become permanent mental states rather than temporary moods. Too little sleep, even if you're otherwise healthy, also increases the likelihood you'll suffer from emotional instability and can worsen or increase the risk of developing serious mental health disorders like clinical depression, anxiety, ADHD, and bipolar disorder. Sleep is such a problem for mood that studies suggest some people diagnosed with depression may not even really have the disease—they might just have chronic sleep deprivation masquerading as depression.

There are a million reasons why people don't sleep well—we could write a whole other book on the topic—but one of the primary drivers of poor sleep is being sedentary. Whether you don't get enough exercise, you sit all day, or you do both, your body stops being able to regulate core temperature properly. This prevents your brain from knowing when it's time for bed, as temperature drops trigger sleepiness. Being sedentary also throws off the body's circadian sleep-wake cycle and ratchets up feelings of stress, sadness, anxiety, and irritability, all of which can make it more difficult for you to fall asleep and stay there. These are some of the reasons why research shows that cardio exercise helps people fall asleep as effectively as taking prescription pills like Ambien.

If you juxtapose facts about sleep and exercise with statistics showing how sedentary Americans are, it's easy to understand why the CDC recently declared sleep disorders a public health crisis in the US. Today, we're more sedentary than we've ever been in all of history, with the average American sitting for up to ten hours a day. That might be less disastrous if most of us were exercising every day (or, alternatively, meditating for each of those ten hours), but we're not: Less than 5 percent of people get thirty minutes of physical activity every day. Instead, most people turn to alcohol, over-the-counter sleep aids, and prescription pills to help them try to sleep at night, when all they really need is a good sweat session or two.

This is not hyperbole—I see it all the time in patients. Take Liza, for example. Liza was in her twenties and working in the fashion industry when she started seeing me. She had acute anxiety, which she attributed to her job, and was using Xanax to sleep at night. But even with the pills, she was getting only about five hours of quality sleep nightly.

When we went through her health history, I saw that Liza had never been anxious or had sleep troubles in high school or college. Of course, she'd also played

sports then and stayed active by walking to classes and participating in the Ultimate Frisbee league on campus in the afternoons. Since graduating and taking a
desk job, Liza was now sitting all day; she didn't think she had time for any type
of physical activity and felt she couldn't afford a gym. While she wanted to blame
her sleeplessness and anxiety on her job, I told her to try exercising five days a
week instead.

After just a month of regular workouts using New York City's local parks as
her gym, Liza's life drastically changed. She started sleeping eight hours at night
and waking up feeling refreshed the next day. Her anxiety began to fade, and she
stopped her occasional use of Xanax to deal with her anxiety. (Note that those
who take antianxiety drugs on a daily basis should work with a practitioner to
slowly wean themselves off the medication to avoid a possible rebound effect, a
worsening of symptoms that can occur when patients suddenly stop taking psychiatric drugs.) Over time, Liza got so much into fitness that she quit her fashion
job to work for a wellness startup. Today, she tells me that she's happier with her
health and her life than she's ever been. Just by adding regular exercise and getting more consistent, drug-free sleep, Liza experienced a State Change.

In my experience as a doctor, no prescription drug, over-the-counter sleep aid,
or supplement like melatonin is going to give you the same quality sleep that
consistent exercise will. Even if you think you don't have any sleep issues, moving more will increase the quality of your sleep and help you feel more energized
and refreshed throughout the day. In Liza's case, her State Change was free, and
helped her unlock a professional purpose in life that she felt more connected to
than fast fashion. It also helped her avoid potential decades of medication and
therapy, costing tens of thousands of dollars, that I see so many patients slide into
in their twenties when they don't adopt the kinds of core actions discussed in this
book to address their emotions, energy, and sleep.

3. Exercise is a requirement—not just a *nice-to-have*—for stress relief.
Modern life is inherently stressful. Most people are dialed into email, text messages, social media, and news around the clock. Our phones are the last thing we
see at night, the first thing we check in the morning, and sometimes what we consult in the middle of the night when we can't sleep or get up to go to the bathroom.

We're constantly connected and go-go-going, whether we're working, managing a family, trying to meet social demands, or, most likely, doing all three.

As a result, most people never experience anything resembling total relaxation at any point during a twenty-four-hour day—or even a seven-day week. Instead, we're always on high alert, causing the sympathetic nervous system (which oversees the body's fight-or-flight mode) to go into overdrive. The result is toxic, driving down immunity, sabotaging sleep, spiking blood sugar, and triggering a perpetual low-grade state of agitation that can lead to depression, anxiety, burnout, and exhaustion.

While other core actions, like which foods you eat and how you interact with technology, can help mitigate stress (see Chapters Six and Seven, respectively), neither provides a direct physical outlet for the cortisol and other harmful neurochemicals most people produce in alarming amounts every day as a result of stress. This is why you *need* exercise—as opposed to exercise being ideal or great if you can fit it into your schedule. You need to be active in order to clear the cortisol, adrenaline, norephedrine, and other chemicals you pump out daily in response to constant connection, stimulation, and stress.

Exercise mitigates stress in other ways, too. Working out forces you to disconnect—after all, it's hard to text, email, or scroll through social media while you're running, doing Downward Dog, or playing tennis. When you're active, you also get you out of your head and into your body, making you more mindful and providing a mental and emotional reprieve away from your repetitive thoughts and emotions. Physical activity also stimulates endorphins, which act like morphine in the body to reduce pain, increase feelings of euphoria, and lower stress.

But not all exercise is created equal: Different forms of physical activity have different effects on our minds and mood. Aerobic exercise, or any activity that increases your heart rate and helps circulate oxygen through the blood, including running, fast-walking, and cycling, produces feel-good chemicals that can increase your sense of well-being for hours afterward. Cardio is also a super-effective and healthy way to distract your mind from your thoughts while helping to expel harmful biochemicals and emotions that can sabotage mood.

Aerobic activity, however, isn't the only mood-boosting exercise. Controlled-movement activities like yoga and tai chi are necessary to ease muscular and mental tension, doing so in ways aerobic exercise cannot, while disrupting the repetitive straight-line movements we do every day (sitting, standing, typing, driving) that can keep our thoughts trapped on play-and-repeat alongside our bodies. Finally, strength-building workouts like weightlifting build muscle mass, which studies show helps to balance blood sugar, lower inflammation, prevent cognitive decline and depression, and boost feelings of confidence and well-being.

My Ultimate Prescription for Mood-Boosting and Flow-Maximizing Exercise

Exercise can accomplish a lot of different goals. You can use it to get fit, build muscle mass, lose weight, improve balance, or increase flexibility and agility. But the ideal exercise program for weight loss isn't necessarily going to help you hone flexibility and balance or help you experience a State Change: Different kinds of physical activity are better suited to different objectives.

Similarly, while doing any type of exercise will improve your mood, if you want to do everything possible to prevent or reverse a mental health issue, adopting some kind of aerobic exercise alongside controlled-movement and strength-building workouts will help you get there faster. I've prescribed the following combination for movement to thousands of patients over the years and seen first-hand how they've benefited by overhauling their mental health and reducing, if not entirely eliminating, their need for antidepressants, ADHD drugs, and pain-killers.

Here's my ultimate prescription for mood-boosting exercise:
- 2 days x 20 minutes of aerobic exercise per week
- 2 days x 30 minutes of controlled movement per week (e.g., yoga, tai chi, qigong)
- 2 days x 20 minutes of strength building per week
- 1 day rest and chill

This is the formula that triggers people to feel better in their bodies, minds, moods, and overall lives and have the State Change they're looking for. But here's the thing: You need all three components to feel really good. I'll explain why over the next several pages, but if you already take spin classes five times per week, for example, or do yoga as your only form of physical activity, you're going to need to weave in a few other things.

Before you start, it's critical to get your mind in the right place. Approaching movement with the proper mindset is the biggest key to success. Here are five mindset shifts that will help make exercise as effective as prescription drugs for mood and mental health:

1. **Be reasonable with your expectations.** If you have moderate to severe depression or anxiety, working out won't completely cure your condition without other interventions, like medication, therapy, and/or dietary changes. But it's an incredibly important part of transforming your mental health, so stick with it.

2. **Be consistent.** In order for movement to treat mental health issues, you need to be active on a regular basis—not just a few times a month or whenever you get around to it. If you think you don't have the time, think again: I promise that you do. Look at exercise as a nonnegotiable part of your day, like eating lunch or commuting to work. This may mean something else in your life has to give, like how much TV you watch or whether you meet someone for after-work drinks or opt for a workout date instead. The best things in life often require a few sacrifices, which, once made, tend to be big upgrades.

3. **Think long-term.** Movement for mood isn't a quick fix—it's a lifestyle. While one workout can boost your mood immediately, in order to treat long-standing issues of depression, anxiety, burnout, ADHD, or brain fog, you need to move your body on a regular basis for months, not just days.

4. **Find what moves you.** In order to make exercise a regular part of your life, it helps to find ways to move your body that you

love to do, not that you force yourself to do. There are lots of different ways to get in a good aerobic workout, do controlled-movement exercises, and build strength. Keep an open mind, experiment a lot, and be persistent, trying new activities for at least several sessions before you rule any out.

5. **Start small—but start somewhere.** For people with depression or low energy, the idea of being active on a regular basis may seem daunting or even impossible. My advice: Start small. Doing something—anything—is better than doing nothing. If you do only ten minutes of activity daily several days a week, that's a life-changing start: It's a lot easier to go from ten minutes a day to twenty minutes a day than it is to go from the couch to forty-five minutes. Just because you can't complete the full prescription detailed here doesn't mean you shouldn't try adding more movement into your life in every way possible.

Twenty minutes of aerobic activity twice a week: Aerobic exercise, which includes running, biking, hiking, swimming, dancing, tennis, the elliptical, and power walking, is the best way to boost the brain's production of endorphins—feel-good chemicals that reduce pain and produce a sense of euphoria similar to the one produced by opioid drugs. The more intense your cardio workout, the more endorphins your body creates.

But aerobic activity does more than provide an endorphin boost. A good cardio workout also distracts you from what's going on inside your head. While working out anywhere will do the trick, if you combine cardio with time spent outside in nature and/or listening to really good music, you can transport yourself to a whole other mental and emotional zone. This temporary break from your perpetual mental-emotional state can set you up to break the cycle more consistently once you experience it.

Aerobic exercise also helps the body detoxify and expel stored emotions and the biochemical cascade they can cause, as we talked about in the beginning of this chapter. By doing cardio, you're literally leveraging your bloodstream, liver, and kidneys to move fear neurotransmitters and stress hormones out of the body and allow more positive emotions and energy to take hold.

If you suffer from chronic fatigue, you may not feel like doing anything active, like aerobic exercise, but the more you don't move, the more tired you'll be. Remaining sedentary locks you in a cycle of exhaustion and lethargy that you have to break with movement in order to have the energy to do more movement. If you feel like you don't have the drive to do cardio, my best advice is to start small. I tell patients with chronic fatigue to do ten minutes of any type of aerobic exercise twice a week—even something simple, like walking up and down a flight of stairs; that's often enough movement to break the pattern.

For most people, however, twenty minutes of sustained aerobic exercise is enough to jump-start their mood while not taking too much time or requiring the kind of motivation or commitment that will dissuade them from doing it regularly. At the same time, if you're someone who likes to run, bike, swim, or do another form of aerobic exercise for longer than that, by all means keep doing what you like. Working out this way for up to an hour six days a week will only increase your fitness, cognitive function, and overall mood and mental health.

If you're struggling to do any type of aerobic exercise, look for forms of cardio that you find fun—there are literally dozens of different types, including everything from doing dance videos to team sports to '80s-style aerobics—and that you can do while listening to music. Research shows that working out to music lifts mood more than exercising in silence, and effectively distracts your mind, allowing you to increase your intensity, effort, and total time. If you're new to exercise, you might want to start out walking around your neighborhood with headphones and your favorite playlist. Personally, whenever I'm struggling with something at work or at home that feels overwhelming and makes my mind spin, all it takes to snap me out of it is a fast walk listening to my workout playlist on Spotify. I find Lady Gaga and Post Malone particularly effective (don't judge me for my music taste), but you do you.

Thirty minutes of controlled movement twice a week: For many of my patients, this component is the biggest lift of all three of my movement requirements. Controlled movement like yoga, tai chi, and qigong (pronounced "chee-guhng") may be gaining ground in Western society, but these types of practices still aren't the norm for most Americans—or even included in federal guidelines for good health. But I'm adamant for several reasons that patients with depression, anxiety, burnout, brain fog, and/or other mood issues make controlled movement part of their weekly routine.

Most people know what yoga is, with more than 55 million Americans practicing the activity at least once in 2020. Tai chi may be less popular, but more and more people, especially millennials, are trying this ancient form of Chinese martial arts that combines slow movements with deep breathing, often known as "moving meditation." Qigong is likely the least well known among the three modalities, but it's similar to tai chi: The practice's simple poses form the foundation of tai chi's more rhythmic movements.

No matter which one you try, it's imperative to do one of these types of controlled movement twice a week for at least thirty minutes. That's because controlled movement accomplishes something that aerobic exercise and strength building cannot: It effectively eases the muscular and mental stiffness we all incur on a daily basis.

When you sit and stare at a screen all day, seven days a week, as most of us do, it creates incredible stiffness in the body and mind. Sitting can cause muscular and mental stress, but so does constantly being stimulated and agitated by media and technology, which is often what we do while we sit—a double whammy for the body and brain. Without enough movement to lubricate your muscles and joints, you literally get shrink-wrapped by your own fascia—the connective tissue surrounding the body's muscles, organs, joints, and nerves. This creates a physical stiffness that compounds the mental and emotional stiffness triggered by sitting all day. What I've seen with my patients is that, when they do some sort of slow, controlled movement, like yoga, tai chi, or qigong, it forces them to stretch their bodies' connective tissue, disrupting the accumulated tension of sitting all day while releasing both mental and muscular stiffness.

Yoga, tai chi, and qigong are also nonlinear movements, meaning they break the constant straight-line spatial world we live in every day by simply sitting, walking, driving, and doing repetitive tasks. With these activities, you stay linear, facing forward, with your head, arms, and legs in a linear or straight line. You don't have to think about how you move, and your body and mind remain on autopilot, thinking the same thoughts, digging the same mental rut, and tasking your muscles and joints to do the same things every single day. Yoga, tai chi, and qigong, however, force your body and mind to move in different directions: You have to make circular or spiral motions, twist your torso, bend upside down, or tense one muscle group while relaxing another. That's very different from how we move 99.9 percent of the time. I've experienced firsthand how nonlinear movement can disrupt the physical and mental rut of linear life, triggering a huge tension release that can help you find a State Change.

Doing rhythmic, controlled movements like yoga, tai chi, and qigong can also create a temporary flow state that, similar to aerobic exercise, takes your thoughts and awareness out of your head and places them into your body. It takes mindfulness and an active mind-body connection to bend upside down, twist outward, do a Downward Dog, or get into Tree Pose, as these movements are hardly customary to everyday living.

But when I talk with patients about doing controlled-movement exercise, I usually hear the same excuses: *It's boring. It's not a workout. I'm not flexible.* If you're making these excuses, however, it's just proof that you need these practices now more than ever.

First off, if yoga, tai chi, or qigong sounds like a snooze, you're certainly not alone. We're all accustomed to being constantly entertained, stimulated, and even jolted awake or alive. Think about what goes on in a typical spin class: You're exerting yourself intensely while listening to blasting music as a teacher screams instructions, dozens of people pump up and down around you, and lights and mirrors flash in the background. When we're at work, we face a constant bombardment of colleagues, calls, messages, emails, to-do lists, and tasks that never lets up. At home and in our off hours, we turn on our TVs and open up our phones, tablets, and laptops for more media and stimulation. What's amazing about yoga, tai chi, and qigong, on the other hand, is that they create the exact opposite environment: There is no hyperstimulation or agitation. It's just you and your body, as you're forced to slow down, be present, and experience a true time of peace. If that sounds uncomfortable, then that's likely a good indicator that these practices are exactly the mental medicine you need.

One of my patients, for example, was entirely opposed to doing yoga, even though it was exactly what she needed to reset her energy, restore her sleep, and get her out of a cycle of burnout that she'd been in for thirty years. At sixty-two, Tori suffered from what I like to call "successful lady boss syndrome": She was a high-powered, high-performing entrepreneur and mother—the kind of woman who seemed to have it all and would do anything for anyone at the drop of a hat. On the flip side, though, Tori had a lot of anxiety, which kept her up at night and interfered with her sleep—which, in turn, caused her to eat everything in sight the next day, since sleep deprivation boosts hunger and cravings. Tori "paid" for this by doing a lot of high-intensity exercise like running, hitting the Stairmaster, and taking spin classes. Slowing down to do yoga was on her no list, she said, because it wouldn't burn enough calories or distract from her endless anxiety.

But given her anxiety, I knew Tori needed yoga more than she needed yet another loud, fist-pumping spin class, so I challenged her to swap out most of her high-intensity workouts for five yoga classes per week for one full month. If Tori hated anything more than yoga, it was saying no to a challenge, so she agreed, warning me that she would likely gain five pounds and be a mental mess the next time she saw me.

Neither happened. When Tori came into my office thirty days later, she was noticeably calmer, happier, and less stressed. She told me that, much to her surprise, yoga had in fact reset her system, physically and mentally, and that she was finally sleeping through the night and not feeling the continually spiraling anxiety that had dominated her subconscious for years. When she measured her belly, she found that she had also taken two inches off her waist: Yoga had lowered her levels of the fat-storing hormone cortisol and helped her to sleep, which regulates metabolism and blood sugar while reducing cravings and appetite. In short, Tori had to commit to slow down—to being in the room and moving with slow purpose rather than frenetic energy—in order to speed up her metabolism and rev up her energy level.

If you've tried meditation in the past and haven't been successful at it, don't worry: Doing yoga, tai chi, or qigong will likely be easier and more comfortable for you than sitting still. And while it may feel funny at first to move in a different way, I want to remind you that there's no "normal" when it comes to movement, even though society seems to have set robotic, linear movements like running and cycling as the gold standard—possibly another reason why we have such high rates of mental health issues in the first place.

When people tell me yoga, tai chi, and qigong aren't a good workout and therefore a waste of time, I say that they're some of the most time-efficient workouts you can do—for your mind as well as your body. It's challenging to have to slow down, pay attention, and bring your awareness into your physical self—for some people, it's a lot easier to go for a fast walk, jog, or read a magazine on an elliptical machine. There are also tons of physical benefits with yoga, tai chi, and qigong, including increasing flexibility, balance, muscle control, and agility, on both musculoskeletal and neurological levels.

If you think you're not flexible enough to do something like yoga, I have a spoiler alert: You don't need to be. First, you definitely don't have to do every position to the degree your instructor or others in the class do: Every body is different, and some of us are flexible in certain ways where others are rigid and vice versa. If you're a runner, biker, or regularly do another type of repetitive exercise and assume you're not flexible enough, that may be because you've shrink-wrapped your connective tissue from so much repetitive motion, meaning you need yoga, tai chi, or qigong more than ever as a counterbalance. And if you truly believe you're inflexible with your body, there's a good chance you're likely also inflexible in your life—another sign you need some sort of controlled movement to help you begin to see and open up new pathways.

Lastly, you don't have to join a yoga studio or martial arts center to take part in some type of controlled movement. If COVID-19 taught us anything, it's that we can find any type of workout video at any time online, usually free of charge. Search YouTube or download an app for yoga, tai chi, or qigong. Be sure to try several different platforms to find the one you like best.

Twenty minutes of strength building twice a week: Most young people take muscle mass for granted. When we're in our teens, twenties, and even thirties, muscle is (or should be) relatively easy to build and maintain. Then, as most people get older, muscle mass starts to decay, lowering immune function and metabolism while increasing the risk of diabetes and bone breaks, alongside dozens of other illnesses and disease. Studies also show people with reduced muscle mass suffer more cognitive decline, depression, and other mental health issues.

In our modern lives, the rapid loss of muscle mass with age has been accelerating. When you're sedentary all the time, no matter how old you are, you prematurely age your body by triggering early muscle loss, effectively turning you into the equivalent of a seventy-year-old when you may be only twenty-five, thirty-five, forty-five, or fifty-five. At the same time, chronic stress alone can cause muscle atrophy, leading to even more physical, mental, and emotional decline.

This is why I tell my patients that they have to find a way to build strength and counteract the muscle loss that's now become a by-product of modern life. You need muscle not only to prevent cognitive decline and mental health problems but also to stabilize blood sugar, lower inflammation, and improve blood flow to the brain. Strength building has also been shown to increase confidence, body image, and mental focus. These are all reasons why research shows that weight training can *significantly* reduce symptoms of depression and anxiety.

To build muscle mass, though, you have to lift weights or do some type of intense resistance work—aerobic exercise alone isn't enough to counter the type of muscle wasting most of us incur by living a sedentary lifestyle. And you can't just lift any weights—you have to lift heavy enough to break down muscle fibers, triggering your body to build those fibers back up again, which is how lean muscle is created. To gain muscle mass, the American College of Sports Medicine recommends doing three sets of six to eight repetitions to the point of fatigue, meaning you couldn't physically do another rep, even if you wanted to. You can complete reps using free weights, weight machines, resistance bands, or even your own body weight. But no matter which method you choose, make sure you're challenging your muscles to the point of fatigue, which requires proper form, especially when using resistance bands or your body weight.

All this isn't to say that you have to join a gym or buy a wildly expensive home setup. You can work out and build muscle mass with just a couple of medicine balls, kettlebells, resistance bands, free weights, or an at-home resistance system like TRX. If you don't own any of these items, you may need to invest in a few things, but most are relatively inexpensive. I have a few resistance bands, ten- and fifteen-pound medicine balls, and several free weights, which I combine to get in a great strength-training workout at home with the help of some online videos. This whole "home gym" setup cost me about $100.

If you're new to strength training or have never done it on your own, it's a good idea to get help so you don't waste your time or, worse, hurt yourself. There are a ton of strength-building tutorials and routines online created by expert trainers who can guide you and help keep your workouts varied and interesting. If you want one-on-one attention, many personal trainers now offer remote online training at reduced rates. You can also ask around at your local gym, fitness center, or YMCA if someone on staff can help you develop an effective strength-building routine.

*

One final note about movement for ending burnout and finding your next level of energy and flow: In our culture, we tend to see exercise chiefly as a means to achieve visual appeal. We care about looking sexy, fitting into the right jeans, or being "summer body ready" more than we care about how we feel in our own skin. But in reality, no matter what we look like, our physical bodies are how we get a lot of enjoyment out of life. Without a physical body, you wouldn't be able to eat really good food, dance in the rain, have sex with someone you love, walk through the woods, swim in the ocean, watch the sunset, or do most of the things that make life worth living. Exercise is a wonderful way to remember that you're a physical person having a corporeal experience on Earth and that your body is as much a part of your existence here as the thoughts and emotions in your mind. While it's easy to forget about your body when you're feeling depressed, anxious, tired, irritable, burned out, or scattered, taking the time to move can reground you in the physical self and remind you of all the joy and bliss you possess in your muscles, bones, and skin.

CHAPTER SIX

Food for Energy, Focus, and Flow

I never thought I'd be a doctor. I thought I was a words girl growing up, not a numbers girl: I did great in English and history and struggled with calculus and chemistry. And didn't you have to be a science and math whiz to be a doc? I was an international relations major in college and had never even considered a career in medicine until I started doing yoga and experienced the State Change in my early twenties that I told you about in Chapter One. That was the trigger for the pieces to eventually fall into place and for me to see myself from a distance. Suddenly, my grandmother's cancer diagnosis, the research I discovered on holistic approaches to prevent cancer in college, the fact that I was a misfit for a legal career, and my messed-up romantic relationship all started to make more sense. My life path opened before me, and the direction I wanted to go was a way I hadn't ever considered before. I realized that I didn't want to be a lawyer or someone who eats toxic food to get through the day or pushes my body to work out just to stay thin. I wanted to feel better. And I wanted to help other people feel better, too. I wanted them to realize what I had discovered—that you actually have more of a choice about whether you feel sick, sad, tired, or anxious all the time than anyone ever teaches you or gives you credit for.

Progress, it turns out, is not linear.

Choosing to become a doctor in my postcollege twenties wasn't easy, though. While I had a ton of credits in French, world politics, and macroeconomics—subjects that definitively don't apply to a career in healthcare—I had zero in biology, physics, or organic chemistry, all of which I needed to ace before I could even apply to med school. This meant I had to go back to my undergraduate university in Philadelphia to earn a postbaccalaureate in premed, a year that essentially amounts to a fifth year of college in time and cost. I crammed my postbac into a single year while also studying manically for the MCAT—the eight-hour standardized test all premed students have to take just to apply to medical school.

I'll be honest: The stress and intensity of that year were almost too much for me. There were days and even weeks when I felt like being back in school to re-graduate with a premed degree three years behind my original class, combined with the pressure I put on myself to get all As so that I could get into a good school, and the fact that I was downright crappy at chemistry, was all too much. I thought about quitting regularly, and I cried to my mom over the phone just as often. I power walked for hours on the treadmill in the claustrophobic basement gym in my building in West Philly while watching Season 1 of *Gray's Anatomy*, hoping that everyone in med school would be as hot, smart, and cheeky as those on the show, despite the fact that, from the looks of things in my postbac class, that was not going to be the case.

The process wasn't over yet: I then had to kill another full year applying to med school and traveling to different universities around the country to interview in person. At that point, I was very much ready to stop wandering around my undergrad campus, feeling stuck in time. I wanted to make money, get out of Philly, and do something during my year before school that would be relevant enough to my future career in medicine to be noticed on my application. After applying for a Fulbright scholarship to India and getting axed in the final round, I started googling research jobs at some of the university medical centers in New York City. I knew the pay wouldn't be great, but it would be a ticket out of Philly and back to my friends in New York—and a chance to try out a new field and figure out what, exactly, I wanted to do with my medical degree.

That's how I came to work for Dr. Mehmet Oz—the same Dr. Oz who now has his own daytime talk show, multiple best-selling books, and a reputation as one of the most influential and controversial physicians in the country. Back in the mid-2000s, though, Dr. Oz wasn't a household name. That's likely why I was able to find his email address openly available on the Columbia University website, where he was (and still is) a professor in the Department of Cardiac Surgery. At the time he was running a research program in integrative and preventive medical protocols for cardiac surgery patients. *Hmm, interesting*, I thought.

I sent him a cold email, volunteering to help him with any possible projects and attaching my CV at the last second in what felt like a Hail Mary, not expecting to hear back.

A few days later, Dr. Oz called me on my cell. Would I help him produce a radio show he was launching out of New York's Lincoln Center recording studios for Oprah? I didn't know what he was talking about. I had no idea that he was already a little famous, and I honestly thought he sounded a bit crazy at first, since I was applying for a research job at Columbia, not to be a radio DJ for Oprah. My dad, who's also a physician, asked if Dr. Oz was legit, but I looked him up again, confirming he had degrees from UPenn and Harvard and was definitely a chair of the surgery department at Columbia. I figured (and convinced my father) that Dr. Oz at minimum was an esteemed leader in his field at one of the country's top medical institutions, therefore making him as legit as I ever hoped to be.

So I took the train from Philly to New York City to interview with him at his office at 168th Street. While I wasn't a math or science whiz growing up—and passing those classes in postbac had taken every ounce of both brain and willpower I'd had—my way with words and writing weren't a waste after all, it turned out: I was well prepared to help produce the first-ever radio show on health and medicine for Sirius XM. I was a super-fast reader, a comprehensive note taker, and a stickler for detail. I was on time and on point. I got the job.

Dr. Oz had never hosted a radio show before—and learning how to host a radio show isn't like learning to make coffee or scramble eggs, where you're pretty much a pro after a thirty-second tutorial. My first three weeks on the show, we recorded hours of practice segments on a variety of subjects, most of which went into the "delete" file, per the *Oprah* producers. When Mehmet started radio, he was a surgeon and an author, not yet a natural talk-show host. We all had to face our own learning curves, it turned out.

During these practice segments, Mehmet talked a lot about his views on the relationship between food and heart disease—a topic he knew well. He told stories from the operating room about how he had to take veins out of people's legs and tie them around their hearts because their arteries were so clogged—something these patients could have prevented by being more proactive about their core actions like eating less sugar, quitting smoking, and exercising consistently. Hearing him speak opened my eyes up to how much I didn't know about nutrition and health. It was also an aha moment for me about my career. I realized I wanted to be on the front end of medicine, helping people fix their health before it was too late, instead of putting them back together like Humpty Dumpty after they were already broken.

A few weeks into our practice segments, Mehmet said something about food with such practiced conviction that it caused me to sit up straight in my seat: *Eating a bagel is like throwing a grenade in your stomach.* When I heard this in the control room, I mentally froze. At the time, a majority of my diet consisted of bagels and bread, after I'd tried to expand into "real food" after my years of protein bars, apples, and coffee. The image of a bagel exploding in my stomach was vivid—and frightening. How could something like a bagel, which nearly everyone I knew ate on a regular basis, be that bad for you? After all, back then, I thought (like most people did) that meat and fat made you fat and low-fat carbs like bread, pasta, pretzels, and bagels were "healthy." But now, a doctor with multiple Ivy League degrees, a prominent position at Columbia, and a regular guest spot on *The Oprah Winfrey Show* was telling me that a staple of my daily sustenance was sickening me in immediate and potentially dangerous ways.

Of course, he was right. What a bagel, along with other refined carbs, like cereal, bread, crackers, pastas, pastries, and chips—even the gluten-free, organic, and/or vegan kinds—do to your blood sugar and insulin can put you on a fast track for chronic disease. As we talked about on page 51, spiking your blood sugar with sugary foods (and refined grains break quickly down into sugar) causes inflammation that not only affects your body but also your brain, sparking possible depression, anxiety, irritability, fatigue, and brain fog. And it's not just processed carbs that can make you sick and sad: It's also all the other processed foods we eat today. That's not just limited to all the traditional junk found on most supermarket shelves but includes gluten-free crackers, keto-friendly protein bars, dairy-free ice creams, grain-free frozen meals, and veggie-oil deep-fried "paleo" vegetable chips.

I have plenty of patients who think they're eating healthy because they're not slugging back sodas or living on chicken nuggets. But plenty of smoothies, fruit-sweetened yogurts, and breakfast cereals contain more sugar than soda, and fast food isn't only sold at McDonald's and Burger King. After producing for Dr. Oz, doing my medical training, and working for ten years in patient care, I've seen how almost all of us are eating fast food on a daily basis, whether it comes from a drive-through window or out of a crinkly bag from Whole Foods.

Nearly everything we eat is processed to be fast and convenient, with added sugar, refined flours, industrial food dyes, artificial flavors, and other ingredients that drive up inflammation and sabotage our physical health and our psyche. Even if you cook at home, if your definition of cooking means using or assembling from mostly premade sauces, boxed pasta, packaged breads, or frozen meals and other processed foods, you're likely still ingesting a lot of sugar and other refined ingredients that can be toxic to the body. The key to healthy cooking is using fresh, whole foods that contain little to no added ingredients and haven't been processed. Cooking with these kinds of foods can take time, though. In short, we live in a world that tells us convenience is more important than health.

The problem with our American diet isn't just what's in it but also what's *not* in it. Processed, packaged, and premade foods are largely devoid of the vitamins, minerals, fiber, healthy fat, antioxidants, and phytochemicals (healthy plant compounds) that can lower inflammation and help fire our bodies and brains to thrive physically, mentally, and emotionally. One reason for this is that processed, packaged foods often contain refined grains, even those that are perceived as so-called health foods, including gluten-free breads, pastas, crackers, and snacks. Refined grains, like white bread, white rice, and most pasta, crackers, and cereal, are those that have been stripped of their fiber and bran. Refined grains include most flours, which are just grains that have been milled and pulverized into a fine dust, making them instantly digestible. Refined flours look like sugar and act like sugar: Since they contain no fat, protein, or fiber on their own, refined grains break down quickly into simple sugar and spike blood glucose, triggering the same dangerous domino effect that sugar does. That's why Dr. Oz compared eating a bagel, rather than a donut, to throwing a grenade in your stomach—it doesn't have to be sweet to be toxic.

Almost everyone I know could use a wake-up call about what they're eating on a daily basis. Getting rid of the sugar and processed junk and examining what you eat to determine whether you might have a food sensitivity, intolerance, or allergy—which at least half of my patients do—are nonnegotiable steps to take if you want to create a real State Change. The patients I see who get off the meds and increase their baseline level of health and happiness are the ones who do this and eat similarly to the way I'll outline in this chapter.

This doesn't mean you'll have to live on kale and nuts to be healthy. You also don't have to wait decades to see and feel what can happen when you start eating for better mental and emotional health. Unlike eating to beat heart disease, fight cancer, lose weight, or tackle another physical ailment, when you eat an anti-inflammatory diet, the mental and emotional results are immediate, with many people experiencing less brain fog, irritability, anxiety, and even depression after only a few days.

If you have kids or spend any time with kids, you already know something about the immediate effects that food can have on emotional health. If my toddler son has ice cream and cookies, for example, he's a screaming, irritable, toy-hurling nightmare. Same if someone gives him the "healthy version" of ice cream and cookies, like a juice box and a cup of gluten-free animal crackers at a party, which contain a combined thirty grams of sugar. He's off the walls, literally high on sugar, and then crashes like a drug addict. It's painful to watch.

While many parents see it clearly in their kids, somehow they don't make the connection to their own bodies. Most of us don't realize how much our diets are sabotaging our psyches. But when you change how you eat and see how that changes the way you feel almost immediately, it's an eye-opening, empowering moment. From there, the more consistently you eat in a way that supports instead of sabotages your mental health, the better it gets, as you gain more clarity, energy, and emotional stability than you may have thought possible.

So, how do you eat to change how you feel and pave the way to a State Change?

When it comes to using food to achieve a healthier mental and physical baseline, the three things that matter the most are (1) balancing blood sugar to prevent inflammation, (2) eating the right types of fat to lower inflammation, and (3) removing foods that you're sensitive to or intolerant of that may be causing even more inflammation. While these three points may sound straightforward, they're difficult to nail in the real world, since most foods we're habituated to eating and encouraged to buy in our local grocery stores spike our blood sugar, don't contain the right kind of fat we need for our brains to function optimally, and can cause sensitivities and allergies. That's why it's important to understand the science behind blood sugar, healthy fat, and food allergies, intolerances, and sensitivities, all of which we explain in this chapter.

I know from working with thousands of patients that simply telling people what to do isn't really effective. People do better when they understand *why* something works. In other words, we change what we eat when we know what a certain food does to our bodies and brains, not when we're given platitudes like *Bagels are bad* and *Kale is good*. So, let's start with the surprising ways that the foods you likely eat on an everyday basis might be sabotaging your mental and emotional state.

How the Foods You're Already Eating Affect Your Energy and Flow

The link between what we eat and how we feel has been researched for years, but few people, even many mainstream doctors, really understand how massive the food-mood connection is. Almost everything you eat either improves or harms your mood, affecting not only your cognitive function but also your propensity for depression, anxiety, brain fog, fatigue, and other mental health issues. Spikes in your blood sugar cause a rapid release of the fat-storing hormone insulin, while simultaneously triggering a flood of other hormones and neurotransmitters to deal with the sugar surge, sending your body and brain on a roller-coaster ride of emotional ups and downs.

Over time, high blood sugar also increases inflammation, a state where your immune system is pumping defend-and-repair chemicals throughout your body and brain. When inflammation occurs in the brain, it's called neuroinflammation, which is short for your brain being on fire because it's sitting in a toxic tea of immune chemicals. How exactly neuroinflammation occurs after a sugary snack or carb-rich meal is pretty interesting. Basically, when you repeatedly spike your blood glucose (glucose = sugar), your immune system responds by activating microglia, the primary immune cells for the central nervous system, found in your brain and spinal cord. As sugar surges through your arteries and veins, these activated cells produce small messenger chemicals called cytokines that, when triggered regularly, cause localized neuroinflammation and can even attack and destroy brain cells. This can lead to cognitive decline, neurodegenerative diseases like Alzheimer's, and mood disorders like depression, anxiety, brain fog, and poor sleep.

Eating too much sugar too often—which most Americans do—affects your mood in other ways, too; for instance, by triggering an overgrowth of bad bacteria in the gut, or microbiome, where your body produces neurotransmitters like serotonin and soothing GABA. When you overgrow certain types of bacteria because you're eating too much sugar, your microbiome can't produce, regulate, or break down neurotransmitters, which can cause or worsen depression, anxiety, brain fog, ADHD, and other mood disorders. Think of it like weeds taking over the grass.

If you're feeling that all the talk of neurotransmitters and microbes is a little abstract, let's focus on how this applies in your daily life: Even if you think you're eating healthfully, you're likely consuming more sugar than you think—and it's likely having a negative effect on your energy and mood. The recommended amount of total sugar per day is thirty-eight grams (no more than nine teaspoons) for men and twenty-five grams (no more than six teaspoons) for women. These numbers represent your maximum *total* sugar intake, including the sugar that's added to processed foods like breads, cereals, snacks, and condiments, as well as natural sugars found in fruit, dairy, and other naturally carbohydrate-containing items, such as vegetables. To put these recommendations into context, a popular all-natural protein bar made from only fruit and nuts contains eighteen grams of sugar per bar, just one serving of the leading brand of yogurt has twenty-nine grams of sugar, and a sixteen-ounce Coca-Cola has sixty-five grams of sugar. Consume any of these items plus even a single meal and you've exceeded the daily sugar max after just a snack—no wonder the average American ingests a whopping seventy-one grams of sugar every day. The symptoms of eating too much sugar include brain fog, fatigue, irritability, trouble concentrating, migraines or tension headaches, acne or frequent skin problems, frequent yeast infections . . . the list is nearly endless.

In addition to added sugar and refined grains, there are two other ingredients found in most of the foods we eat that inflame our brains and mess with our microbiomes: refined vegetable oils and industrial food chemicals.

Vegetable oils may have the word *vegetable* in them, but there's nothing healthy about these fats, as evidenced by the fact they're in almost all processed foods—which make up approximately 70 percent of the average American diet. These are cheap, industrial oils that have been chemically extracted from seeds, grains, or legumes and include the very commonplace canola oil (rapeseed oil), safflower oil, corn oil, peanut oil, soybean oil, and palm oil. Vegetable oils are also commonly heated to high temperatures during processing, causing them to oxidize, which produces harmful free radicals, and treated with chemicals to improve their flavor or appearance. We're not saying you need to be fearful of your food, but it pays to be picky about the kinds of vegetable oils you consume, which we'll show you how to do later in this chapter.

Eating more healthy fat may be in favor right now, but the kind of fat found in vegetable oils can hurt your body, not help it. In my opinion, "healthy" fat means choosing omega-3s over omega-6s and prioritizing fatty cuts of seafood and well-sourced, grass-fed meat that's less inflammatory than the industrial-raised, grain-fed norm. When it comes to vegetable oils, most contain high amounts of omega-6 fats, which can increase inflammation in the body. While your body needs some omega-6 fat to function, the problem is we're eating way too much of it and not enough of the essential omega-3s, which help lower inflammation. To put this in perspective, the average American ratio of omega-6 to omega-3 fats hovers somewhere around 20:1, when it should be no higher than 4:1—which was the average ratio one hundred years ago, before refined vegetable oils existed. Our modern-day crazy-high consumption of omega-6s is almost all due to refined vegetable oils. One study from the United Kingdom estimates that the average adult consumes eleven pints of cooking oil per year (mostly in the form of cheap vegetable oil), chugging the equivalent of nearly six bathtubs full of the toxic stuff over a lifetime.

Your ratio of omega-6s to omega-3s matters so much because omega-6 fats in excess produce inflammation and compete with your body's ability to use omega-3 fats. One particular omega-6 fatty acid, known as arachidonic acid (AA), is especially problematic because, in excess, it causes a cascade of biochemical effects that harm brain cells, ratchet up neuroinflammation, and reduce your body's ability to use serotonin, the feel-good neurotransmitter. That's right: Even if you produce plenty of serotonin, your brain can't use it if you're inflamed. What's more, you already know from Chapter Three that your brain is approximately 60 percent fat, 20 percent of which is made up of AA and the omega-3 fat docosahexaenoic acid (DHA). But if you consume too much refined vegetable oil, which breaks down into AA, your brain will start to make more cells with this harmful omega-6 fat, driving up neuroinflammation and leading to unhealthy cellular function. This, in turn, can significantly increase your likelihood of issues like depression, anxiety, brain fog, and even bipolar disorder, while also boosting your risk of memory loss and even Alzheimer's.

Finally, most processed foods contain industrial food chemicals, including preservatives, emulsifiers, artificial flavors, fake food dyes, and synthetic sweeteners. You can also find pesticides, hormones, and highly carcinogenic compounds known as PFAS, or per- and polyfluoroalkyl substances, in animal products and conventionally grown (non-organic) produce, as well as in packaged foods. In fact, there are upward of fifteen thousand known chemicals in our food supply, many of which don't even have to be listed on a product's label, per the FDA, and some of which have never been tested for safety, according to the Environmental Working Group. Common food additives can kill healthy bacteria in our microbiome, triggering low-grade neuroinflammation, along with anxiety, depression, brain fog, and behavioral problems, according to studies. Some chemicals are even outright neurotoxins, meaning they can kill brain cells or interfere with their function, leading to ADHD, brain fog, irritability, sleep problems, anxiety, and depression.

I'm not trying to scare you with this research, but I think it's important to understand how the foods so many of us eat every day are anything but "safe," even if they are "generally recognized" as such. They are inflaming our brains and potentially keeping us locked in a permanent pattern of feeling sad, anxious, irritable, confused, or tired. Now let's look at what you can do to change that pattern—not in months or even weeks but in several days' time.

Eat to Be Happy and Healthy

If you're worried that you have to stop eating everything that tastes good and brings you joy in order to overhaul your mental health and have a State Change, I promise you that's simply not true. I know from my own experience that when I finally started eating to fuel my body and brain rather than just eating what I thought was healthy or would make me thin, I was shocked at how much I enjoyed food—probably for the first time since I was a kid, with no fear of gaining weight. No ups and downs in energy. No insane levels of pickiness. I found a new framework for how to choose foods that would nourish my body, and I could immediately feel the difference, not just in how my body responded but also in my mind. When I started eating this way, my relationship with food changed for the better. Now I love food. I love cooking and eating out. I love trying new foods from around the world and using food as a compass on vacations to experience new places. Today, my husband and I watch hours of cooking shows, like *Top Chef*, *No Reservations*, and *Chef's Table*, geeking out on culinary culture. We are both living proof that there are a ton of delicious foods that your mouth will thrive on as much as your mind and body will.

WHAT ABOUT SALT?

Although many of us spent our childhoods hearing how salt is evil, sugar is a far bigger dietary devil than sodium. While a chronically high-salt diet can increase blood pressure, which can be especially problematic for those dealing with existing heart conditions such as congestive heart failure or who are at a greater risk of developing heart disease, sugar will derail your overall heart health more quickly and effectively than excess sodium. The best way to deal with salt is to eliminate or reduce your intake of processed foods, which are the primary source of excess sodium in the standard American diet. This means that if you're cooking most of your meals with real whole foods, you can break out your salt shaker without worry.

The principles that I follow when it comes to choosing and preparing foods are what we call at Parsley Health a *plant-based paleo diet*. Eating plant-based paleo relies on two core actions:

1. **Eat *Lots* of Plants,** especially whole vegetables, which should make up the majority of what you eat every day.

2. **Cut the Refined Crap,** by which I mean the top four toxic foods that hijack our minds and mood: added sugar, refined grains, refined oils, and industrial food chemicals.

We'll take a deep dive into these four toxic food groups in just a minute, but I first want to make it crystal clear that a plant-based paleo diet doesn't mean restricting, denying, calorie counting, or dieting. When you start eating plant-based paleo, you get to consume a ton of super-yummy foods, including fresh fruits, vegetables, nuts, seeds, beans, legumes, spices, meat, seafood, and whole grains. These are the foods, when consumed in their whole, unprocessed form, that balance blood sugar, increase circulation, support heart health, boost the microbiome, improve immune function, and reduce neuroinflammation. And yes, you can eat meat and animal products on a plant-based paleo plan. It's not vegan—it's just plant-focused.

The kind of foods you eat when you're plant-based paleo will also help your brain become more elastic—meaning your mind will be more cognitively flexible and able to think about things in multiple ways—and more plastic, meaning it can rebuild and rewire itself, helping you recover more quickly from stress, recall what you learn, master new skills, and prevent or reverse mood disorders. Increasing brain elasticity and plasticity on a plant-based paleo diet can help you make faster decisions, manufacture the right neurotransmitters at the right times to cope with stress, clean your brain's neurological trash at night while you sleep, and better adapt to life's inevitable changes. In other words, consuming more plants and the right kinds of fat, fiber, and proteins—and eating fewer processed foods, added sugars, unhealthy fats, and other toxins—can biohack your brain to help you become not only smarter but also more mentally and emotionally resilient.

A plant-based paleo plan is a powerful way to supercharge your flow, whether you're suffering from a major mental health disorder or have a low-grade case of depression, anxiety, irritability, brain fog, or fatigue. I compare eating plant-based paleo to getting to base camp at Everest: You can't climb the mountain without making it to base camp first, and you can't fix your mood until you change your diet. For some people, eating plant-based paleo is the one thing that takes them all the way to the top, effectively reversing their mood problem. For others, eating plant-based paleo removes a roadblock that's prevented them from reaching the summit, allowing them finally to make progress toward reversing or stabilizing their mood disorder with the help of medications and therapy. No matter where you're starting from, food can be the key to better mental health.

WHAT ABOUT A KETO DIET?

The ketogenic diet may be all the rage right now, but it's not the way I think everyone should eat for optimal health. Achieving true ketosis, a state when your body burns fat for fuel instead of carbohydrates, requires you to get at least 75 percent of your total calories from fat for days, which can be difficult to sustain. For some people, keto can backfire, too, causing them to gain weight, increase unhealthy levels of LDL cholesterol, and, for those with certain genetics, potentially cause long-term cardiovascular damage. The way I look at the keto diet is that it's not a lifestyle but a tool that a plant-based paleo eater can use occasionally to boost metabolism, lower blood sugar, and clean up dead and dying cells in the body. This is what I call doing *a keto sprint*. We'll talk more about how, why, and when to do a keto sprint on page 145.

What, exactly, does eating plant-based paleo mean? Unlike other biohackers in my field, I don't define paleo as consuming only what ancient paleolithic people ate before the advent of agriculture. As a working mom, I can tell you that that's just not practical or realistic. Many healthy foods, including things like big, leafy stalks of kale, olive oil, and walnuts, are byproducts of modern-day agriculture. What matters more than avoiding foods that did not exist in the days of ancient humans is avoiding produce and animal products that are grown or raised with pesticides, hormones, industrial grain feed, and other toxins. Perhaps even more important, it matters that we avoid agriculturally produced foods that leave the farm or ranch and are then processed or refined, such as veggie chips, hot dogs, and frozen pizza.

I also don't define paleo as dogmatic, meaning you can still follow the plan whether you want to be a vegan, vegetarian, or omnivore. What's more important than whether you eat meat is if you include sources of toxin-free, high-quality protein in your diet, whether that's from organic almonds, lentils, and quinoa, or wild salmon, grass-fed beef, and pasture-raised chicken and eggs. Personally, I eat a mix of eggs, high-quality seafood, grass-fed beef, and veggies, while avoiding poultry and pork for ethical reasons and because it's very hard to find sustainably sourced versions of those animals. That said, what works for me might be different than what works for you for ethical, health, environmental, or accessibility reasons. What I hope you and I will have in common after you read this book is what we largely don't eat: refined packaged and processed foods, added sugars, and industrially farmed animals and produce.

It's important to prioritize organic produce and grass-fed or pasture-raised animal products whenever we can: As we covered on page 126, toxins found in conventionally raised fruits, vegetables, and animal foods can seriously mess with your brain's ability to function. At the same time, I understand not everyone has access to these foods or can afford them—unfortunately, governmental subsidies given to the corn and soy industries make processed, refined foods and food additives much less expensive than healthy, whole foods. I would encourage everyone to make an effort to eat organic or grass-fed whenever possible, with the understanding that you should never let the perfect be the enemy of the good. If you can't find organic spinach or afford grass-fed steak, don't throw in the towel: You'll still reap a ton of benefits by dropping a standard American diet of refined sugar and grains for a plant-based paleo plan, even if it's made up of mostly conventionally raised foods.

Eleven Amazing Ways to Eat Plant-Based Paleo

When it comes to eating to support your body and brain, there are ten groups of foods to focus on—and one big "paleo" trend to avoid. Learning to prioritize the right foods will help stabilize your blood sugar, reduce neuroinflammation, rebuild your microbiome with healthy bacteria, and change your mental and emotional outlook for the long term.

1. Make 50 percent of your plate green at every meal.

If you don't change your current diet in any way other than making sure at least half of your plate consists of leafy green vegetables, you'll still significantly improve your physical and mental health. That's because leafy green vegetables are extremely potent sources of vitamins, minerals, antioxidants, phytochemicals, and fiber, without all the calories, carbohydrates, and added sugars found in most foods. Piles of research show that consuming more green vegetables can help reduce neuroinflammation, regulate blood sugar, lower toxic buildup, feed healthy gut bacteria, and improve blood and oxygen flow to all your organs, including your brain—all of which can overhaul your mood, energy, mental function, and sleep in quantifiable ways.

Leafy green vegetables include the obvious—spinach, kale, arugula, romaine, collards, mustard greens, etc.—along with those that people don't necessarily think of as "leafy," like broccoli, brussels sprouts, bok choy, and cauliflower (which belongs to the same family as kale). Leafy green vegetables *don't* include any versions of these plants that have been commercially processed into broccoli tater tots, brussels sprouts doodles, packaged kale chips, cauliflower crackers, or spinach pasta. The leafy greens on your plate should look like they came out of the ground, not off an industrial conveyor belt. Cooking at home usually solves that problem—it's harder to add a bunch of sugar and chemicals to fresh spinach or kale in your own kitchen.

Try to eat leafy greens during your first meal of the day—it will help balance your blood sugar and recharge your brain. If you like traditional "breakfast" foods, even if you eat them later in the day because you're intermittently fasting (see page 143), make a spinach omelet, layer arugula over smashed avocado and quinoa, or blend kale with berries, nut milk, almonds, collagen powder, and ice for a morning smoothie.

2. Upgrade your oils to these three brain-friendly fats.

You got the memo on page 125: refined vegetable oils increase neuroinflammation and interfere with omega-3 absorption and function. Eliminating packaged, processed, and premade food—even takeout, since restaurants usually use cheap vegetable oils—will cut out a lot of refined fats from your diet. What to use instead? My three favorite fats are extra-virgin olive oil, cold-pressed coconut oil, and ghee, or clarified butter that has a higher smoke point than regular butter and almost no lactose (milk sugar). Here's why these three are my top picks:

Extra-virgin olive oil (EVOO) is not a refined vegetable oil. It's made by pressing olives once through a cold or stone press. EVOO is more flavorful than regular olive oil, which is often chemically processed and refined, and EVOO contains a ton of nutrients, like vitamins E and K. EVOO is also rich in many different antioxidants, including some shown to work similarly to ibuprofen, reducing inflammation, and certain polyphenols, or plant compounds, that studies show can actually deactivate genes that trigger inflammation. In addition to lowering inflammation in the brain, EVOO may also help fight the kind of brain-based plaque that causes Alzheimer's disease, while improving blood flow, regulating blood sugar, and reducing oxidative damage to cells. For all these reasons, research shows consuming more EVOO can help combat depression, anxiety, brain fog, and ADHD.

Like EVOO, cold-pressed coconut oil isn't refined but pressed from coconut meat without any additional processing. Coconut oil is a buzzed-about health food for many reasons, but what I like about it is that it's rich in medium-chain triglycerides (MCTs)—a type of saturated fat that heads immediately to your liver, where it's either used as energy or turned into ketones. Ketones are fatty acids that can cross the blood-brain barrier and provide an alternative fuel source to glucose for hungry brain cells. And feeding the brain fat, not sugar, has been shown to improve cognitive function, boost mood, and reduce the risk of neuro-degenerative disorders like Alzheimer's. Research also shows that coconut oil's unique combination of MCTs and antioxidants can help lower neuroinflamma-tion, mitigate symptoms of depression, treat anxiety, limit fatigue, and help fight sleep disorders.

Ghee, or clarified butter, is another great addition to your kitchen cabinet and mental health arsenal. This rich-tasting butter derivative is one of the best dietary sources of N-butyrate, a short-chain fatty acid that helps feed and heal the cells that line the gut. When your gut lining is well nourished, it can help lower neuro-inflammation, brain fog, and depression via that powerful gut-brain axis—the two-way highway between our microbiome and mind that makes the microbiome our "second brain." Ghee is also good for high-heat cooking since it has a higher smoke point than other oils and has little to no lactose (milk sugar) or the dairy proteins casein and whey, making it tolerable for those who are lactose intolerant or have a dairy sensitivity or allergy. If you want to make your own ghee, you can gently melt butter and skim off the white protein foam, leaving the clarified fat below.

3. Eat your brain-boosting Bs.

Some people develop neuroinflammation and mood disorders for one reason: They're not getting enough critical B vitamins in general or are low in one of the eight essential Bs we need for good physical and mental health. Here's the thing, too: It's really easy to be B-deficient. Since our bodies can't store B vitamins, we have to consume them through food on a regular basis. Eating too much sugar or refined grains can deplete your B stores, as can too much stress, alcohol, or caf-feine, all of which increase the rate at which you pee out your Bs. Certain medications can also prevent optimal B absorption, including birth control pills, as can medical disorders like celiac and Crohn's disease. And certain gene variations like MTHFR can make it more difficult to absorb and use Bs if you aren't getting the right kinds (see page 78).

While you can take B supplements (more on what to look for when choosing a B supplement on page 199), the best way to regularly absorb the nutrients is through food. B vitamins in general are found in a ton of foods in the plant-based paleo plan, including legumes, nuts, seeds, dark leafy greens, eggs, and animal foods, but not all eight Bs are present in all foods. The most critical Bs for mental health are B_{12}, folate, B_5, and B_6, so it's important to make sure you're consuming specific foods that contain these specific nutrients.

B_{12} may be the most critical B vitamin for mental health—and also the one that people are most likely to be deficient in. Low B_{12} is associated with depression, anxiety, brain fog, and fatigue. That can be a big problem if you're not eating enough meat, seafood, or dairy, since B_{12} is found only in animal products like beef, tuna, salmon, chicken, eggs, milk, and yogurt. Breakfast cereal, nutritional yeast, and many dairy alternatives are now fortified with B_{12}, but science shows that we absorb nutrients better from foods that naturally contain them, since those foods include a range of other vitamins, minerals, antioxidants, and phytochemicals that increase the nutrients' bioavailability. If you're vegan and have been struggling with mood issues for some time, you may want to consider consuming a small amount of seafood, beef, or dairy in order to get B_{12}. Clams, sardines, and salmon are some of the best sources of B_{12}, and are packed with anti-inflammatory marine omega-3 fats, which are also challenging to get enough of on a vegan or vegetarian diet.

Another way to help mitigate symptoms of depression is the B vitamin folate, also known as B_9, so much so that the nutrient is seen as a possible treatment modality. Research shows that folate can improve cognitive function, alleviate anxiety and brain fog, and improve overall mood, in addition to helping with depression. Legumes like beans and lentils are high in folate, as are asparagus, beets, dark leafy greens, eggs, citrus fruits, broccoli, nuts and seeds, and liver.

Two other B vitamins—B_6 and B_5—don't get the same amount of buzz that

B_{12} and folate do when it comes to mental health, but both are essential for our cognitive function and mental and emotional health. B_6 helps convert the amino acid tryptophan into serotonin and plays a key role in suppressing inflammation. Foods highest in B_6 include chickpeas, tuna, salmon, chicken, potatoes, and bananas. B_5, or pantothenic acid, can also be called the "anti-stress" vitamin because it helps regulate production of neurotransmitters and hormones that influence our calm level. Top sources of B_5 include mushrooms, sunflower seeds, chicken, tuna, avocado, potatoes, and eggs.

Right now, you might be thinking there's no way you can keep track of all these B-rich foods to make sure you're getting your daily dose. I get it. That's why I like whole eggs (not egg whites or liquid eggs): They contain all eight B vitamins and are a good source of high-quality protein, omega-3 fats, and other micronutrients. They're also relatively inexpensive, pair well with leafy green vegetables, and are easy to cook with, even if you're a neophyte in the kitchen. I recognize that some people have egg allergies—if that's you, turn to the other sources of Bs listed above.

4. Consume more brain-friendly fats.

Americans are eating more fat than we ever have before, studies show. But we're not consuming the right kind of fat for our mental health. You can even be on a keto diet and eating a ton of fat, but if it's coming mostly from beef and chicken, deli meats, or all those "keto-friendly" bars, chips, cookies, and other snacks, you're likely deficient in omega-3s, which help lower neuroinflammation and balance that critical ratio of omega-6 to omega-3 fats.

Not all omega-3 fats are created equal. As we talked a little bit about earlier in this chapter, there are big differences between the plant omega-3 ALA (alpha-linolenic acid), found in foods like nuts, seeds, soy, and avocado, and the marine omega 3s, EPA and DHA, which are found primarily in seafood. While ALA is considered an essential fatty acid, it's not biologically active until it's converted into EPA and DHA. But our bodies can only convert 5 percent of the ALA we consume into EPA and a dismal 0.5 percent of ALA into DHA.

That conversion rate becomes a big problem if you, like most Americans, don't consume enough seafood. EPA and DHA are imperative to basic brain function and health and can help prevent and even treat depression and other mood disorders. Both EPA and DHA can travel through the blood-brain barrier and actually repair cells, lower neuroinflammation, and make it easier for serotonin to move throughout the brain. Studies show that people with a high intake of DHA also have a 50 percent lower chance of anxiety. Additionally, marine-derived omegas play a critical role in cognitive development and function and help to prevent neurodegenerative diseases like Alzheimer's.

For all these reasons, I believe marine omega-3s are the most critical fat you can eat for your overall physical and mental well-being. But few of us are actually eating enough of them. While marine omegas are in lots of seafood, EPA and DHA are found predominantly in fatty fish like salmon, herring, tuna, mackerel, anchovies, sardines, and flounder. Americans aren't eating much of these fish, or any other seafood for that matter: We consume less fish and shellfish than any other industrialized country, and we're taking in less than half the recommended two four-ounce servings per person per week for general health. Adding insult to injury, when Americans do eat seafood, they're mostly consuming shrimp, which is low in EPA and DHA and is often contaminated with antibiotics, pesticides, and other toxins.

Seafood also contains mood-boosting vitamins B and D that can be difficult to get from other food sources. I recommend taking a fish oil supplement, especially if you're vegan or vegetarian or don't eat any fish. Be sure any supplement you take is made from a high-quality source of fish oil, not algae or other plant sources; however, the body absorbs up to nine times more EPA and DHA from seafood than it does from supplements. If you're strictly vegan or allergic to fish, you'll have to really double down on algae and unrefined plant-based fat sources. The biggest mistake I see people make in these categories is that, unintentionally, fat simply gets eliminated from the diet, handicapping everything from mental and cardiovascular health to gut and hormone balance.

5. Feed your body's microbiome.

One of the best ways to support the cooling and clarifying of your brain is to eat foods that help promote a healthy population of bacteria in your gut, otherwise known as your body's microbiome. The microbiome is ground zero for your body's neurotransmitter production and also headquarters to control your mood and the levels of inflammation in your brain.

Every food on a plant-based paleo plan will help increase the health of your microbiome by feeding your gut's good bacteria—you can literally set it and forget it. But if you're dealing with digestive problems, brain fog, and/or other mood issues, you'll want to give your microbiome a boost by consuming more fermented foods like kimchi, miso, pickled vegetables, tempeh, low-sugar yogurt, and fermented coconut milk. Fermented foods contain live strains of bacteria known as probiotics that replace the healthy gut microbes most people kill every day through a cocktail combo of stress, sugar, processed foods, alcohol, chemicals in our food supply and the environment, antibiotics, and other prescription drugs.

Studies show that increasing the amount of good bacteria in your gut improves the immune system, helping your body better regulate neurotransmitters like serotonin (needed for good mood) and melatonin (needed for sleep) while lowering inflammation throughout your body and brain. The result is that consuming foods that contain probiotics—i.e., fermented foods—can help limit depression, anxiety, and irritability, improve sleep, reduce fatigue, boost memory, and even increase cognitive function. Probiotics have also been shown to help treat autism and obsessive-compulsive disorder.

The effect that probiotics have on the brain can be major. Studies show that people who regularly consume probiotics can even change areas of the brain associated with mood, according to brain scans. One study from the University of California, Los Angeles, for example, found that women who ate yogurt twice a day for just one month had brain scans showing they were calmer than a control group of women who didn't eat yogurt, after both groups were shown images of facial expressions displaying happiness, anger, sadness, and other acute emotions. Researchers say they were shocked by how sharp the contrast between the two groups was, and they credited the effect to the ability of probiotics in yogurt to produce compounds that actually change brain chemistry.

Probiotics are so imperative to mental health that researchers have even coined the term *psychobiotics* to describe the brain-altering effects that good microbes can have on our minds and mood. Consuming probiotics in fermented foods has also been shown to aid weight loss, improve digestion, lower "bad" LDL cholesterol, and reduce the risk of allergies, infections, digestive conditions, and eczema and other autoimmune disorders.

So far, science has shown that two probiotic strains can be especially beneficial to mental health: *Lactobacillus* and *Bifidobacterium*, which are found in most yogurt and kefir. Since the bacteria in these foods help to digest milk sugar, both unsweetened yogurt and kefir can be tolerable for those who are lactose intolerant. But if you have a dairy sensitivity or allergy, I recommend eating yogurt and kefir made from fermented coconut milk, which is also high in probiotics. Kimchi, miso, non-genetically modified tofu, and raw, unpasteurized sauerkraut are other good sources of probiotics—just keep in mind that heating these foods over 115 degrees Fahrenheit can kill their live bacteria.

Although kombucha has become a popular fermented beverage, I'm not a fan of consuming it as a source of probiotics. I love it as a carbonated treat on occasion, but most commercial brands contain too much sugar and too few probiotics to be part of your daily routine.

Probiotic supplements that actually contain live microbes—I'll show you how to find the best ones in Chapter Eight—should be part of any biohacker's mental health kit, but you shouldn't rely on supplements alone. Research shows that fermented foods have a greater diversity of bacteria than supplements. They also contain enzymes that help the gut better break down nutrients in other foods.

6. Reset your taste buds' preferences with nature's candy.

Sugar is in almost every packaged, processed, and premade food we eat, whether it tastes sweet or not. The ubiquity of sugar, combined with the amount the average American consumes per day (a massive 17 teaspoons), has desensitized our taste buds. This means we now need more and more sugar in order for food to actually taste sweet to us—one reason why food manufacturers have consistently increased the sugar content of food over the years. Today, extra sugar is in everything from salad dressings and bread to takeout Thai food and pizza. Even worse, natural sugar levels found in foods like fruits, vegetables, and dairy don't even taste sweet to most Americans anymore.

Here's the good news: It's totally possible to reset your palate so that you actually taste sugar like your grandparents or great-grandparents did. The best way to do this is with a thirty-day elimination diet, detailed on page 147, in which you eliminate all added sugar and processed foods (most of which contain added sugar) for one month. The effect is eye-opening: My patients at Parsley who do this elimination tell me after three weeks that they can taste food in a way they haven't before, or that they haven't since they were kids, when watermelon was considered a dessert. From there, a handful of organic strawberries or a few slices of mango can feel like a sugar explosion in your mouth—in a good way. When you reset your taste buds, nature's candy is more satisfying than an ice cream sundae.

7. Slow the metabolic burn with nuts and seeds.

Packed with B vitamins, minerals like magnesium, antioxidants, and other micronutrients, nuts and seeds help slow how quickly foods in your meal spike your blood sugar. That's because nuts and seeds are some of the few foods that are rich in healthy fat, fiber, *and* protein, all of which work together to mediate the body's blood sugar response (and thereby inflammation).

Here's how it works. Let's say you eat a bowl of rice or quinoa topped with vegetables, which, on its own, probably sounds pretty healthy. While it is, for the most part (you're doing a great job on your phytonutrients and fiber!), this meal is still mostly made up of carbs, with almost no fat and not much protein. You need more fat and protein to prevent your blood sugar from rising quickly in response to the naturally occurring carbs in these grains and veggies. So, if you were to add just a handful of crushed almonds, chopped macadamia nuts, or pumpkin seeds to your bowl, along with a drizzle of extra-virgin olive oil, your blood sugar won't spike as quickly, which in turn will mitigate inflammation in your body and brain. Nuts or seeds will also make the dish more filling and provide a better source of slow-burning, lasting energy.

The benefits of nuts and seeds go far beyond blood sugar. They've also been shown to lower oxidative stress and improve blood flow, helping improve mood and cognitive function while countering depression, anxiety, brain fog, and fatigue. One large nine-year study of more than twenty-six thousand people found that those who ate walnuts every day—the nut with the highest levels of ALA omega-3s and antioxidants—had a 26 percent lower depression score on average. Those who regularly ate nuts of any kind also had more optimism, energy, hope, concentration, and a greater interest in their everyday activities.

Certain nuts have different distinct benefits for our mood, too. For example, Brazil nuts, which provide 1,000 percent of your recommended daily dose of selenium and up to 33 percent of the daily dose of magnesium per one-ounce serving, may help counter anxiety and depression, in part because both minerals are extremely calming. On the other hand, pumpkin seeds are an excellent source of tryptophan—they contain more per one hundred grams than turkey—which the body converts into serotonin.

There are a few things to be cautious about when it comes to eating nuts and seeds, however. First, peanuts aren't actually nuts but rather legumes that can contain aflatoxin, a mold known to increase inflammation, cause food allergies and autoimmune problems, and trigger serious health issues for anyone with a mold allergy. If you love peanuts, they're still a better choice than anything sugary or processed, but try to substitute other nuts when possible. The same goes for cashews, which have more carbs than other nuts—nine grams per ounce, which is more than double the amount found in walnuts, pecans, and macadamia nuts.

I would also encourage you to opt for raw nuts and seeds over the roasted varieties whenever possible. That's because roasted nuts are often overcooked, causing them to lose their nutrient value and oxidize their fats, which produces harmful free radicals. Energy bars loaded with nuts tend to be bound with sugary dates or drenched in other sweeteners, whether natural or not, that also outweigh the benefits.

8. Load up on magnesium.

This essential mineral is responsible for more than three hundred biochemical reactions in the body, including helping to create new proteins, repair genetic material, convert food into energy, and regulate neurotransmitter production. Without enough magnesium, you can develop problems with your thyroid, sleep, metabolism, and mood, among dozens of other ailments.

When it comes to mental health, I like to think of magnesium as nature's

Xanax. My patients who actively work to eat more magnesium often tell me they feel a greater sense of calm and relaxation after a few weeks. On the other hand, people with low magnesium levels have been shown to have a higher incidence of depression, anxiety, sleep difficulties, and brain fog. Some researchers even point to magnesium deficiency as the root cause of many cases of subclinical depression and believe the mineral should be more widely used as an adjunct treatment alongside antidepressants.

Despite how critical magnesium is to our overall health, at least 50 percent of all Americans are deficient in the mineral. One reason is because food today contains less magnesium than it did several decades ago due to industrial farming practices that have largely depleted our soil of key nutrients. Some scientists even call this widespread deficiency of magnesium in plants an urgent problem.

For these reasons, it pays to be deliberate about eating foods high in magnesium, just as we need to do with B vitamins. The best food-based sources of magnesium are many of the same foods essential to a plant-based paleo plan, including pumpkin seeds, chia seeds, spinach, almonds, dark chocolate, black beans, edamame, quinoa, and tuna (look for products by Safe Catch or Wild Planet, both of which are lower in mercury than conventional brands).

9. Eat mushrooms to evolve your neural pathways.

While more and more research shows that psychedelic mushrooms can transform our mental health, which we'll talk about in Chapter Nine, I want to focus here on the types of shrooms you can find in the supermarket. I strongly believe everyone should be consuming mushrooms at least twice a week since the evidence is only growing that fungi can alter our mood in incredible ways.

The first thing to know is that mushrooms aren't like other plants: Fungi are the forest's original internet superhighway, working to connect the roots of all types of plants so that they can share nutrients and information that make them more resistant to possible pathogens and disease. When it comes to cognitive health and mood, lion's mane mushrooms—a type of white, stringy shroom that looks like a lion's mane or sea anemone—have been shown to lower neuroinflammation, stimulate the growth and differentiation of brain cells, counteract memory loss, and improve how well your hippocampus, which is the part of the brain responsible for your emotional responses, works. Research has also found that lion's mane mushrooms, which you can find at natural food markets like Whole Foods or for sale online, can act similarly to antidepressants while also limiting anxiety. If you cook lion's mane mushrooms long enough, they develop a texture similar to meat and are both tasty and filling.

Another shroom with mood-boosting benefits is the reishi, which you may have seen marketed in powders, tinctures, and teas. But you can also eat these mushrooms—find them fresh or dried online—added to soups, broths, and smoothies (they're especially good in grain-free baked goods and dairy-free shakes made with dark chocolate). Studies show reishis can stop the growth and spread of cancer cells while improving immune function, but when it comes to our mood, they've also been shown to help control blood sugar, limit fatigue, and reduce the symptoms of depression.

While reishis may be a bit harder to find, oyster mushrooms, available at most supermarkets, have also been shown by research to reduce inflammation, protect against cognitive decline, and boost brain function. This common mushroom is also loaded with antioxidants and other nutrients and may lower cholesterol, according to animal studies.

10. Whole grains are good grains.

If you're not sensitive to grains, I have no problem including small portions of whole grains like brown rice, quinoa, amaranth, oats, and millet as part of a plant-based paleo plan. The only caveat—and it's a big one—is that they have to be whole grains that you can see, not ones that have been ground up into flours, made into processed pastas, or otherwise disguised in refined foods. Additionally, grains shouldn't form the majority of any meal. Instead, prioritize veggies, nuts, seeds, legumes, seafood, and animal protein. If you eat too many grains, even the healthy whole kind, you can still develop blood sugar issues and increase neuroinflammation, undoing what you want to accomplish by eating plant-based paleo. Aim to consume no more than one-half cup of grains per meal for a max of two meals every day.

11. Forget packaged "paleo" products.

The paleo diet has been trendy for years, and a lot of food manufacturers have capitalized on the buzz by marketing foods as paleo when they're anything but. If you buy a "paleo" food that's vacuum-sealed or has a long ingredient list, there's nothing healthy or paleo about it: More than likely, it contains added sugar, refined grains, refined oils, and/or food chemicals. Focus instead on whole, healthy foods and leave the packaged "paleo" junk on the shelf.

Why, When, and How to Use Fasting to Improve Your Energy and Flow

Intermittent fasting is all the rage right now—and for good reason. Studies show that not eating between dinner and lunch the next day (basically skipping breakfast to achieve a sixteen-hour overnight fast) can lower inflammation, reduce oxidative stress, increase human growth hormone production, boost blood-sugar regulation, speed metabolism, improve cellular repair, fire up brain-cell growth, aid in weight loss, help prevent cancer, and even increase longevity. To get these kinds of benefits, most research suggests restricting your calorie intake to an eight-hour window—for example, eating only between 12 p.m. and 8 p.m.— giving your body a sixteen-hour respite from having to deal with metabolizing food, half of which time you're asleep. During this metabolic break, your body will access stored fat as an energy source and will more adeptly repair cellular damage. For these reasons, I intermittent fast a few days a week and recommend that my patients try it, too. I find intermittent fasting improves my focus, energy, and mental clarity. I also don't think it's that difficult to do, especially once you get accustomed to it—after all, we're just talking about missing breakfast, which, for the majority of Americans, who are already overfed from a caloric perspective, isn't a big deal. That said, intermittent fasting isn't for everyone—women who are pregnant or those with a history of eating disorders, for example, will want to avoid it. And some people find more benefits than others; intermittent fasting is a practice that, along with a healthy, plant-based paleo eating plan, can give you added benefits, but it's not a miracle cure.

I could spend more time on intermittent fasting, but a more substantiated approach when it comes to our physical and mental health is something called prolonged fasting, which means not eating any calories for two to five days. While that may sound extreme at first blush, it's really one of the most natural things we can do. Humans have evolved to be able to withstand days without food, going back through all those years when we couldn't find our next meal ready and pre-wrapped at any restaurant, supermarket, or deli. Today, though, most of us continually bombard ourselves with calories, which the human body hasn't evolved to handle like a perpetual tidal wave. Instead, our constant food consumption has caused widespread rates of weight gain, obesity, metabolic disorders, chronic physical disease, and chronic mental illness.

Not only is eating around the clock not good for your physical or mental health, there are also several distinct biological advantages to punctuated periods of prolonged fasting. Research shows that when we go without food for at least forty-eight hours, it forces our bodies to blow through our glucose and glycogen stores, which triggers our bodies to start burning fat for fuel. Burning fat for fuel results in the production of chemicals called ketones, which have been shown to spur the production of new immune and stem cells, while prompting other cells harboring harmful or dysfunctional molecules to self-destruct in a process known as autophagy.

One of the most eminent researchers of prolonged fasting, a biologist named Dr. Valter Longo, compares the effect to taking cargo off a plane in order to lighten the ride and make your body fly more efficiently. I think of it like spring-cleaning: If you don't let your liver clean out its energy stores, or you don't allow your cells to get rid of all their junk, stuff just accumulates. Imagine every closet, drawer, and cabinet in your house were full, and junk was covering the floors and filling up every room. How well would you be able to function in your own house?

Prolonged fasting—by which I mean at least twenty-four hours without calories—has also been shown to slow cellular aging, reduce inflammation in the body and brain, improve blood sugar levels, trigger weight loss, and even help prevent and treat cancer, according to research. Specific to mental health, periodic prolonged fasting has been shown to slow, stop, or, in some patients, reverse depression, anxiety, brain fog, and fatigue, while increasing feelings of emotional well-being.

The good news is that you don't have to (and should not!) prolong fast every week or even every month to hack your mind, mood, and cellular age. Instead, I recommend doing either a *fasting sprint* or *keto sprint* at most once or twice a year—or, at the very most, once every season. These are simply two different ways to complete a prolonged fast and reap all the physical and mental health benefits listed above.

What's the difference between a fasting sprint and a keto sprint? A fasting sprint is when you fast for five consecutive days, consuming nothing other than water—no calories from food or liquids. A keto sprint is when you follow a strict ketogenic diet, getting at least 75 percent of your total calories from fat, for five consecutive days. Consuming this much fat forces your body to go into ketosis, when your brain and body start burning ketones for fuel instead of sugar, mimicking the effects of fasting even though you're still eating.

A keto sprint appears to provide the same benefits as a fasting sprint, but since you can consume food and caloric liquids, it's oftentimes easier and more realistic for people to do. As a doctor, I don't often recommend a water-only fast, but I do a keto sprint at least once a year, and I recommend some of my patients do, too. Note, however, that you need to get at least 75 percent of your total calories from fat for a keto sprint to produce the benefits of a prolonged fast. Otherwise, many people who believe they're eating keto don't actually go into ketosis since they don't consume enough fat, regardless of their low carb intake. Even if you eat ridiculously few carbs on this fast, if you consume too much protein and not enough fat, that protein will be converted into carbs, kicking you out of ketosis.

No matter whether you do a keto sprint or a fasting sprint, be aware that undertaking any type of prolonged fasting is difficult and isn't for everyone. At the same time, the physical and mental benefits of prolonged fasting for some make it highly worth the effort. And the good news: You only need to prolong fast once or twice every year, with a maximum of no more than once every season. There's no research supporting the hypothesis that regular prolonged fasting is more beneficial—i.e., more is not better. In addition, if you do decide to prolong fast for the first time, or on a semi-regular basis, you should work with your doctor to make sure it's not negatively affecting your nutrient levels or overall health. And if you have a history of an eating disorder, uncontrolled blood sugar disorder, or are pregnant, breastfeeding, or trying to get pregnant, fasting is not for you at all—period. No matter your health issues, always consult with your doctor before undertaking any type of fast.

Why fast for five days instead of two? While research shows you get some benefits after forty-eight hours of water only, it takes most people at least one or two days after they stop consuming food to enter a fasted state. That's because most of us are eating so much all the time that our bodies need a day or two to burn through all our glycogen stores before we really begin to fast.

KICK OFF YOUR FAST WITH MY MORNING GLORY COFFEE

If you struggle to intermittent fast for a full sixteen hours or are looking for a boost when you do a keto sprint, my recipe for Morning Glory Coffee can help stop hunger cravings, balance your blood sugar, and feed your brain to give you more focus and energy. The recipe uses coconut or MCT oil, so it's dairy-free and vegan. These oils also have benefits that butter doesn't: The medium-chain triglycerides (MCTs) found in both bypass the liver so they're not stored as fat and help produce ketones that feed the brain to boost cognitive clarity. At the same time, the oil won't kick you out of a fat-burning state. A pinch of cinnamon adds a flavor kick and helps stabilize blood sugar further.

Ingredients

2 cups organic, fresh brewed hot coffee

1 tbsp organic coconut oil or MCT oil

¼ tsp of cinnamon

Place all ingredients in a high-speed blender and blend for one minute. Note that the heat of the coffee will melt the coconut oil, so you don't need to melt it beforehand. Recipe makes two servings.

Whenever you do a keto sprint, it's important to continue eating plant-based whole foods as part of your plan. There's a misconception that keto means eating all the cream cheese, pepperoni, and sausage you can find—or that you can load up on packaged, processed keto bars and fat bombs all day. But doing so won't bring you the benefits of a keto diet or keto sprint. Focus instead on plant-based fats like olive and coconut oils, along with avocado, nuts and seeds, seafood, and grass-fed animal meats in moderation. Be sure to keep eating plenty of dark leafy greens and other low-carb vegetables. For specific macronutrient counts and suggestions, look online—there are a ton of trusted sources where you can find out more information on how to follow a strict plant-based ketosis diet.

Kick-Start Plant-Based Paleo with a Thirty-Day Elimination Diet

An elimination diet is one of the most powerful things you can do for your body and brain. I don't know a single person who hasn't felt remarkably better after completing the elimination diet we recommend to most new patients at Parsley, especially those struggling with depression, anxiety, sleep difficulties, fatigue, and/or brain fog. It's easy and free to do, it doesn't require a prescription from a doctor, and it's one of the best ways to determine if what you eat has been making you feel sick or suboptimal, physically, mentally, or emotionally.

Going on our elimination diet at Parsley accomplishes three major feats:

1. You reset your palate, reducing how much sugar you need in order for food to taste good.

2. You significantly reduce any cravings for packaged, processed, or premade foods that contain added sugar, refined grains, refined oils, and/or food chemicals, all of which can sabotage physical and mental health.

3. You can successfully determine if you have a food sensitivity, intolerance, or allergy, each of which is a separate condition that can cause or exacerbate mood issues.

If you've heard about elimination diets or even tried one in the past and still aren't convinced of their efficacy, I want to clear up a few misconceptions. First, eliminating the food groups I suggest—processed foods, those with added sugar, all gluten, and all dairy—is *not* equivalent to starvation.

I have new patients who say to me, *Oh my god, cheese is my life raft*, to which I respond, *If cheese is your life raft, we have bigger problems than I thought*. I'm not asking you to live off of sticks and berries for thirty days straight. I want you to eat really delicious things, like eggs and avocado for breakfast; a big salad with beans, blueberries, mushrooms, nuts, and olive oil for lunch; and salmon with stir-fried veggies for dinner. An elimination diet is an amazing opportunity to learn how to eat really yummy foods while biohacking your body and brain in one month's time.

Plenty of my new patients tell me they've tried giving up all sugar, processed foods, gluten, and/or dairy, but that doing so had no discernible effect on their overall well-being. But here's the thing: You can't eliminate these foods for a few days or even one week and expect to see big changes—if anything, if you've been used to consuming these foods for a long time, you may experience withdrawal symptoms and feel worse at first, for several days, than you did before. What's more, if you have a sensitivity or allergy to a food, your body has been producing antibodies to that food, and it can take a few weeks to clear these from your system. This means you won't really know how you feel off of a food until week three or four without it, when your body stops producing inflammation in response to it. I've seen everything from acne to constipation to joint pain to brain fog go away by the fourth week of an elimination diet, but not usually in the first week or two.

Before I detail exactly how to do an elimination diet, let's talk about why it's important and where you might have come across the concept before. Oftentimes, elimination diets are prescribed to people who think they may have a gluten sensitivity, dairy intolerance, or outright allergy to these ingredients or other common trigger foods, like soy, corn, or grains. But the idea of food sensitivities, intolerances, and allergies isn't well understood by most people. While gluten allergies and dairy intolerances may seem more commonplace these days, studies show that up to half of people who believe they have a food allergy don't actually have one—many have a food sensitivity or intolerance instead. Knowing which one you may or may not have will help you manage and eradicate any physical or mental symptoms you may be feeling as a result.

Much of the difference between a food sensitivity, an intolerance, and an allergy comes down to the kind of immune response your body does or does not produce after you eat a food.

When you have an allergy to a food, your immune system produces antibodies called IgE, short for immunoglobin E. *Antibody* is a funny word, but antibodies are simply proteins that our immune system uses to attack and defuse harmful substances, including foods, that invade the body. These antibodies produce an immediate reaction, usually within minutes or even seconds of your eating a food, that can trigger hives, itching, and instant digestive issues like nausea, vomiting, and diarrhea. Food allergies can be life-threatening, and while many people are born with them, you can also develop them later in life, even as an adult.

So what's a food sensitivity, and how is it different from an allergy? A food sensitivity occurs when the body produces antibodies called IgG, or immunoglobulin G, which are the body's "memory" antibodies. These antibodies will "remember" a food you ate in the past as an invader and appear in the body several days later when you encounter the same food again, often leading to more subtle symptoms—like fatigue, digestive issues, headache, brain fog, and skin problems—than food allergies do. If you have a food sensitivity, the response is usually low and slow—this is why so many people miss food sensitivities or incorrectly attribute their symptoms to the wrong foods or other issues. For example, if you have a sensitivity to casein, a protein found in dairy, you may experience an eczema flare-up two to three days after having ice cream or milk. This can make it tricky to connect the two, unless you cut out dairy entirely for a few weeks then reintroduce it to see if you have a reaction.

Finally, some people have what's called a food intolerance, which means your body simply doesn't tolerate a food very well, not that you have a specific immune response to it. Food intolerances can produce many of the same symptoms that food sensitivities do, including digestive issues, brain fog, and headaches. Intolerances are caused by many different things. Your personal composition of gut bacteria may not be able to break down a certain food, for example, or you may be chronically stressed, which dampens our digestive activity. You may also lack an enzyme necessary to break down a certain food. For example, 65 percent of all adults are lactose intolerant, meaning their bodies don't manufacture lactase, the enzyme necessary to digest lactose, the sugar found in milk. Being lactose intolerant, marked by symptoms of digestive issues like bloating, gas, and diarrhea, is different than having a dairy sensitivity or allergy, which means you're sensitive or allergic to whey and/or casein, the proteins in dairy.

While you probably know already if you have a food allergy, many people with food sensitivities or intolerances—around 50 percent of all my patients—have no idea that a certain food is inflaming their body and brain and potentially sparking or worsening feelings of depression, anxiety, fatigue, brain fog, irritability, or other mood issues. Dairy and gluten are the two most common foods that can cause these problems for patients. You likely know if you have a wheat allergy, which means you're allergic to foods that contain wheat. That's different from celiac disease, an autoimmune reaction to gluten, the protein found in wheat. Around 1 percent of Americans have celiac disease, which is also different from a gluten sensitivity.

Some elimination diets ask you to exclude up to a dozen different foods, including eggs, soy, corn, legumes, peanuts, nightshade vegetables, caffeine, alcohol, and/or all grains. While this kind of strict elimination diet has merit at times, most people don't need to be this restrictive unless they've already completed our core elimination diet for at least thirty days, which excludes all processed foods, added sugars, gluten, and dairy. I find that highly restrictive elimination diets are difficult to do, and many people give up on them before they see results or can determine if a certain food is problematic for them.

While testing does exist for food sensitivities, cutting out all inflammatory foods for at least four weeks' time is the best and most effective way to tell if a food is affecting your physical or mental health. That's because food sensitivity testing is often inaccurate and can pick up things that aren't really long-term sensitivities. At Parsley, we usually reserve food sensitivity testing only for those who have been diagnosed with an autoimmune disease or have chronic inflammation that we haven't been able to source. If they do test positive for a food sensitivity, we still ask them to complete an elimination diet to see whether removing the food alleviates their symptoms or whether they can tolerate small amounts of the item without issues. Finally, there is no way to test for a food intolerance: Doing an elimination diet is the best way to diagnose one.

How to Do an Elimination Diet

A thirty-day elimination diet is one of the most critical things you can do in order to fine-tune the core action that has one of the biggest impacts on our energy and mood: what we eat. Here's what you need to know:

ELIMINATE THE FOLLOWING
FOODS FOR THIRTY DAYS

- **Processed foods:** This means cutting out almost everything that doesn't look like it came directly from a farm. If it comes in a box, bag, wrapper, or package, there's a good chance it's processed. There are important exceptions, like nut butters and milks that don't contain any added sugar or other additives, frozen vegetables and fruit, and olive and coconut oils; when selecting those, check the ingredient list closely to make sure that they do not contain added sugars, preservatives, or other chemicals. One of the best ways to tell if a food is processed is to read the ingredient list: As a general rule of thumb, if a food contains more than one ingredient other than salt, herbs, and spices, it likely shouldn't be part of your elimination diet. And remember that some foods with few ingredients, like deli and cured meats, canola oil, and soybean oil, can still be super-processed.
- **Added sugars:** If you stop eating processed foods, you'll cut out almost all added sugars. But you still need to be vigilant about reading ingredient labels of everything you eat, just to make sure it includes no added sugar, since sweeteners are almost everywhere these days. This isn't just about processed

white sugar, either; you'll also want to avoid adding things like honey, maple syrup, or agave to food and drinks, along with artificial sweeteners like Splenda and Equal. Stevia, monk fruit, and other all-natural zero-calorie sweeteners are fine in moderation when used to sweeten whole foods or drinks, like coffee, tea, yogurt, or oatmeal. But if you're consuming these sweeteners in packaged, processed foods or combining them with refined grains to make cakes, muffins, or other nutritionally poor snacks, you're defeating the purpose.

- **Gluten:** Gluten is a protein found in wheat, rye, barley, and triticale (a cross between wheat and rye). It's found in hundreds of foods, even those that you would never think of, like some ketchup, broth, soy sauce, deli meat, egg substitutes, blue cheese, and flavored coffee. Avoiding processed foods will help you get most of the gluten out of your diet, but you should also steer clear of whole rye, barley, bulgur, couscous, wheatberries, durum, farro, spelt, KAMUT, einkorn wheat, farina, brewer's yeast, oats (unless labeled gluten-free), and anything made with malt, all of which contain gluten.

- **Dairy:** Like gluten, dairy is insidious in our food supply, showing up in all sorts of foods you would never think of as containing cow product, including canned tuna fish (which may contain casein) and restaurant steaks (which are often cooked in butter). When you buy foods in bags, boxes, or wrappers, always check the ingredient list to be sure they don't contain milk, cheese, milk fat, buttermilk, butter, yogurt, or any dairy derivatives, like whey, casein, lactose, caseinates, or hydrolysates (and if they do contain any of these dairy derivatives, you're not buying a whole food but something processed, since no food in its natural state contains a derivative).

EAT THE FOLLOWING FOODS FOR THIRTY DAYS

- **Vegetables** will make up the bulk of your diet, and anything you find in whole form in the produce or freezer aisle is fair game, including artichokes, asparagus, avocado, broccoli, brussels sprouts, cabbage, celery, cucumber, eggplant, raw garlic, kale, onions, rutabaga, spinach, tomatoes, zucchini, collard greens, arugula, lettuce, potatoes, sweet potatoes, squash, parsnips, and beets. While a functional doctor may advise that some people with autoimmune conditions eliminate certain veggies, this is a good place to start.

- **Fruits** are another cornerstone of the elimination diet. Focus on low-sugar fruits, particularly berries, apples, and pears, and be careful about eating too many high-sugar items like mangoes, oranges, and bananas. What's more, prioritize eating these fruits whole, baked, or frozen in simple smoothies made with low-sugar protein powder or unsweetened non-dairy milk. Avoid dried fruit, which is super-high in sugar, along with commercially made smoothies and premade fruit concoctions like acai bowls, most of which are masquerading sugar bombs.

- **Unsweetened nut butters and nut milks,** including almond, cashew, and coconut.

- **Grass-fed or pasture-raised animal products,** including beef, bison, chicken, lamb, turkey, and eggs.

- **Seafood,** including salmon, halibut, mackerel, mussels, herring, anchovies, and sardines. To find low-toxin, sustainable cuts of seafood, consult the Monterey Bay Aquarium Seafood Watch guide at seafoodwatch.org.

- **Beans and legumes,** including chickpeas, kidney beans, and lentils.

- **Nuts and seeds,** including almonds, hazelnuts, pecans, walnuts, sunflower seeds, pumpkin seeds, flaxseeds, chia seeds, and coconut meat.

- **Gluten-free grains,** including quinoa, millet, amaranth, buckwheat, brown rice, wild rice, and gluten-free oats.
- **Herbs and spices,** including sea salt, black pepper, basil, cinnamon, cloves, dill, garlic, ginger, oregano, paprika, rosemary, thyme, and turmeric.
- **Oils and fats,** including virgin coconut oil, extra-virgin olive oil, sesame oil, flax oil, red palm oil, and coconut butter.
- **Condiments,** like lemon juice, sauerkraut, and raw organic apple cider vinegar.
- **Beverages** like water, coffee, chicory root coffee, and tea.

WHAT TO EXPECT DURING THE ELIMINATION DIET

Some people experience withdrawal symptoms the first few days of an elimination diet, including mild headaches, fatigue, and cravings. Try to push through them—this is a sign that your body needs to get these foods out of your system. After the first week, these symptoms should subside, replaced by a heightened sense of well-being.

HOW AND WHY TO REINTRODUCE FOODS

One purpose of an elimination diet is to determine if a sensitivity or intolerance may be causing physical or mental symptoms. If you stop the diet after thirty days and go back to eating all the gluten, sugar, and dairy you want in one fell swoop, you won't be able to identify whether either is a trigger food for you. Instead, you need to reintroduce one new food at a time, one week at a time. Let's start with gluten.

To reintroduce gluten after you finish the elimination diet, begin by eating one serving of an unprocessed or minimally processed food that contains gluten, such as farro, whole-wheat bread, or whole-wheat pasta. Wait forty-eight hours before you eat gluten again, writing down whether you experience any symptoms like digestive issues, headaches, acid reflux, depression, acne, irritability, lethargy, anxiety, or skin rashes. If you don't have any symptoms, try eating gluten again another two days later, repeating the forty-eight-hour cycle for one full week. At the end of one week, if you haven't experienced any symptoms, you likely don't have a sensitivity or intolerance to gluten. If you do have symptoms, you likely have a gluten sensitivity or intolerance and should continue to avoid foods that contain it.

After you reintroduce gluten for one full week, start to eat dairy, repeating the same method by eating an unprocessed or minimally processed dairy product at forty-eight-hour intervals for another full week. If you did determine you have a possible sensitivity or intolerance to gluten, though, be sure to avoid consuming any while you reintroduce dairy.

What about reintroducing sugar and processed foods? I've got some bad news: There's never a good time or reason to reintroduce added sugar. Even though you can't have a clinical sensitivity or intolerance to sugar, if you start eating a ton of it again, it can cause many of the same symptoms as a food sensitivity or intolerance will, including digestive illness, mood changes, sleep difficulties, skin issues, and headaches. The same goes for processed foods. What's more, now that you've reset your palate and don't need as much sugar or crave processed foods as much, try to keep them out of your diet as much as possible. This doesn't mean you can never eat ice cream, chips, crackers, or sausage again. Instead, I would encourage you to view added sugar and processed foods as occasional treats, not everyday sustenance.

MEAL SUGGESTIONS ON AN ELIMINATION DIET

BREAKFAST

- Morning Smoothie: Blend 1 cup unsweetened almond milk, ⅓ cup blueberries, ⅓ cup raspberries, 1 tbsp almond butter, 1 cup baby spinach, and 1 serving plant-based protein powder with ice or water as desired.
- Chia Seed Pudding: Cook 1 cup unsweetened coconut milk, 3 tbsp chia seeds, 1 tsp vanilla extract, and a dash cinnamon over medium heat until it gels. Refrigerate for several hours before serving.

- Millet Porridge: Cook ½ cup millet with ⅔ cup water until it forms a porridge. Mix in 2 tbsp coconut butter, dash cinnamon, 1 tbsp flax seeds, and ½ cup raspberries.

LUNCH

- Super Green Salad: Chop the leaves from 3 to 4 stalks kale and combine with ½ avocado, a handful chopped red cabbage, a handful chopped celery, a handful chopped cucumber, and 1 sliced, grilled chicken breast. Mix and dress salad with 1 tbsp olive oil, 1 tbsp lemon juice, 1 tbsp apple cider vinegar, sea salt, and black pepper.
- Grains Salad: Combine ½ cup cooked quinoa, ½ avocado, a handful chopped red onion, a handful chopped artichoke, and 1 tbsp sunflower seeds. Mix and dress salad with 1 tbsp olive oil, 1 tbsp lemon juice, sea salt, and black pepper.
- Order a salad from your favorite takeout restaurant without any cheese, croutons, wontons, bacon, salad dressing, or any other dairy, gluten, or processed foods or meats. Dress with olive oil and vinegar.

DINNER

- Salmon & Greens: Serve 1 filet baked salmon with a side of Super Green Salad (see above).
- Roasted Chicken: Serve roasted chicken with sauteed spinach and roasted sweet potatoes (flavor with olive oil, not butter).
- Turkey and Veggie Sauté: Heat olive oil over medium. Add garlic and chopped carrots, and sauté until the carrots start to soften. Add ground turkey and sauté until cooked through. Serve with mixed greens or steamed veggies of your choice and optional side of grain.

SNACKS

- **Veggies and Hummus:** Make homemade hummus: Blend 1 can rinsed, drained chickpeas with 2 tbsp olive oil, 1 tbsp lemon juice, 4 tbsp water, and sea salt and black pepper to taste. Serve as dip with sliced carrots, celery sticks, broccoli, snap peas, and/or bell pepper.
- **Roasted Nuts:** Roast your own nuts: Spread 1 cup almonds and 1 cup walnuts on a baking sheet, drizzle with olive oil, sprinkle with sea salt and 2 sprigs rosemary, finely chopped. Bake for 15 to 20 minutes at 350 degrees and cool before serving. Serving size is a quarter cup.
- **Celery & Almond Butter:** Spread 1–2 tbsp almond butter in sliced celery sticks and sprinkle with sea salt and cinnamon if desired.

CHAPTER SEVEN

The Universal Addiction Killing
Our Minds and Draining Our Mood

D on't get up. Don't move. Just reach out your arms. Can you touch your phone? Or your smartwatch, tablet, TV, laptop, or desktop? Without getting out of your chair or taking a single step?

Thought so. Most of us are tethered to technology every waking hour and within an arm's reach of our devices at night. This constant connection to tech, while convenient, is killing our emotional and mental health in more ways than we think. (Hint: It's not just about the blue light.)

Before I go into how our universal tech addiction is causing us a host of mental health issues, I want to tell you about Leah. Leah came to see me four years ago, when she was twenty-four, to help with her treatment for a rare auto-immune disorder she had had since she was a child. As it turned out, taking care of the disease was the easier part of Leah's diagnosis: I was able to identify several food allergies and an overgrowth of yeast that were triggering the prob-lem, which we effectively treated, putting her condition into remission within eight weeks.

But as her physical symptoms started to subside, Leah's anxiety became more pronounced. Feeling uneasy and stressed out wasn't new for Leah: She had devel-oped anxiety as a kid when her physical health first began to regress. The stress of being a "sick person" so young in life, in addition to the years she had endured frustrating interactions with the medical system, had left her understandably discouraged, burned out, a bit jaded, and in her words, "uncomfortable in my own skin" and "always worried something is going to happen." This mindset was a low-grade issue at times and on other occasions was all-consuming, causing her to suffer crippling insomnia, panic attacks, and exhaustion. Over the years, she had seen a psychiatrist, who had prescribed her antidepressants and anti-anxiety drugs, but none of the medications ever helped her feel any better. When the coronavirus pandemic began in 2020, it comprised a new trigger and Leah started to spiral down and feel worse again.

When we met again in the fall of 2020, Leah wasn't taking any psychiatric drugs, and I asked her whether she wanted to start again: Her anxiety was peaking, and I didn't want her to suffer. She had adopted almost every other core action she could to combat anxiety: She was eating a low-sugar, plant-based diet, exercising regularly, and supporting her nutrition with a targeted regimen of supplements. I wasn't sure what else we could do, and I wanted her to be safe. But Leah was adamant about not taking prescription drugs again, not because she was against them but because they had never worked for her, and her psychiatrist agreed. So we started to look at what else she could do.

Racking my brain for what could help, I began asking Leah deeper questions about how she spent her time, digging back into the initial assessment we give all Parsley patients, which she had filled out a few years ago. I asked her if she wore a smart device that tracked her activity and sleep, hoping that we could use the information these wearable devices provide to give us more insight. When we started talking about her technology habits, I began to realize just how much time Leah was spending on digital media—in addition to the time she spent in front of a screen as part of her full-time job as a hospital emergency department administrator, we're talking more than five hours per day, scrolling through Facebook, Instagram, TikTok, CNN, Buzzfeed, and other platforms, all of which had become a bottomless pit for her. That's when it hit me that Leah didn't just have an autoimmune disorder: She also had an addiction to technology.

Unlike my older patients who, similar to me, had had an analog childhood without handheld devices permanently attached to their fingers, Leah had a tech addiction that had persisted for years: She hadn't known a moment in the past thirteen years, or since she was fourteen, when she hadn't been attached to her phone, a time frame which happened to sync up with when she developed anxiety.

With those dots connected, I urged Leah to do a thirty-day detox from all social media and news media, during which time I told her she really shouldn't look at these platforms at all. Astonishingly Leah agreed, which surprised me since this was a big ask for someone with her degree of addiction.

Two months later, Leah came back to see me at Parsley. Before we sat down together, I reviewed the Parsley Symptom Index (PSI) she had filled out in advance of our appointment (you can find the modified version of the PSI beginning on page 32). I was pleasantly surprised to see that her symptom score on the PSI was significantly lower than it had been before her previous appointment, especially in relation to mental health markers for anxiety and depression. I asked her if she had actually completed the thirty-day digital detox we talked about, and not only had Leah done it, she told me that she'd also continued it past the one-month mark, avoiding all news and social media apps for nearly two months total. The result was that her anxiety, which had been sky-high at our last visit, had all but receded, along with a noticeable reduction in her depression and overall stress level. Despite the fact that a pandemic was raging and the US political landscape was chaotic, putting nearly every one of us on edge, Leah was as calm as a cucumber, at least compared to how she'd felt two months before. In some ways, she was an entirely different person: She had had a powerful State Change. What's more, she had this State Change not after altering multiple core actions but after altering only one: her relationship with technology.

Leah's story was also a big aha moment for me. I'd watched her suffer from anxiety for almost four years, and nothing had sustainably worked—not drugs, foods, exercise, supplements, or changes to her sleep hygiene. What turned the key for Leah and unlocked her massive state change was transforming how she used digital media—that and that alone. I had always thought of changing a patient's tech habits like smoothing the proverbial icing on the cake—something that could help alleviate their mental health issues but could never end their condition altogether. But now I know that tech addiction can be the cake itself, or the sole factor driving a person's persistent anxiety, brain fog, attention disorder, insomnia, or excessive fatigue.

I wish I had been able to identify Leah's tech addiction earlier. But these days, it's totally normal to spend hours a day inhaling digital media and living virtually through our phones or computers, because that's what we all do. In this sense, most people are addicted to technology to some degree—and especially to digital media like social networks and online news. We've been brainwashed and peer-pressured by tech companies into believing that these constant streams of information are not only normal but also necessary in our lives, even though they're making us sick. But most of us don't want to acknowledge just how bad our tech habits are, because to admit that would be to confess to swimming upstream vigorously in a harmful experience we've all allowed ourselves to be swept away by.

While estimates vary of how many people actually have an unhealthy dependency on tech, along with what that looks like in an age when nearly every American has to use a connected device for work or out of similar necessity, other data suggests how widespread our collective problem has become. We know, for example, that the average American spends eleven hours a day staring at a screen, which includes smartphones, tablets, TVs, laptops, and computers. In those eleven hours, we spend approximately 2.5 hours on social media, which accounts for five years total of each of our lives, while we're touching our smartphone more than 2,600 times per day. That's how embedded technology is in our lives.

One thing I want to make clear: At no point do I think that anyone can walk away from technology or throw out all their devices. Tech serves a lot of beneficial purposes, and those purposes are only increasing in the digital age. But that's why it's so important to make sure that you're maintaining a healthy, not harmful relationship with tech. It's up to you and you alone whether you decide to consume digital media or allow it to consume you.

Nowadays, I spend a lot of time thinking about how tech hurts not only our physical health—contributing to back and neck problems, eye strain, and our country's sedentary crisis and obesity epidemic—but also our mental health, including my own. Like most Americans, I can spend at least eleven hours a day staring at a screen, maybe even more since the COVID-19 pandemic. The moment I finish work emails, video calls, Slack marathons, PowerPoint decks, and Excel models, I often turn to a screen at home to do an online workout, catch up on Instagram, or watch a TV show to unwind. But whenever I spend this much time with devices, I feel absolutely exhausted, even though I've been sitting all day. My eyes feel like they're swimming inside my head, I'm terribly foggy, and my mind generates this low-grade buzzing. My husband will ask me questions, and I'll start to answer, then trail off and start looking at my phone again.

For me, these effects aren't consistent. I can reverse the mental fatigue and brain fog I feel from tech by taking a day completely away from screens. And when I do so, I feel a minimum 20 percent happier, by my own estimation. Twenty percent! And I'm not someone who suffers from depression. For those with mood disorders, the difference could be even more significant.

I haven't always had all the answers. When I started medical school in 2007, the first iPhone came out, and I immediately got one. Not all my peers felt the same way. Most continued to use flip-phones or BlackBerries, some of which didn't have internet access and none of which had the ability to power apps that create an endless geyser of information, like all smartphones do today. With my iPhone, I created Facebook and Twitter accounts, downloaded early-gen news apps, surfed the web wherever I was, thought I was cool when I was using Firefox early, and even began to think about how these platforms could transform medicine.

In 2009, while still in medical school, I bought a domain name, Cureatr.com, and started brainstorming with a friend in my class what a modern medical communications app could look like. By the time we graduated in 2011, the two of us had hired a developer from San Francisco and were building a digital messaging and communication platform designed for healthcare providers. By this point, I had been fully bitten by the tech bug and never stopped to think about how the digital world might hurt our health, only how it could improve it.

Knowing what screens do to my mood has forced me to take a hard look at how I consume tech—and how I can limit it. As CEO of Parsley Health, I know that digital media is necessary for my job—I can't opt out completely—but I don't want to spend the next forty-plus years of my life looking at screens for up to eleven hours a day. For these reasons, I've had to be resourceful and find ways to limit my tech consumption, which I'll share with you later in this chapter.

No matter how you embrace tech (I embrace it a lot) or what you believe about its benefits (I believe tech has incredible capabilities and possibilities to transform our future) or how much your work or social life depends on digital devices (my work entirely depends on digital), you can reboot your relationship with tech so that it's not interfering with your mental health. I've had to do this, and Parsley has helped hundreds if not thousands of patients do it, too.

But in order to reboot your relationship with tech, you first need to understand what tech is actually doing to your body and brain. Otherwise, it's really hard to fathom the impact that something so culturally ingrained and normalized in society is having on you. That's why I want to start with the science.

You Use Technology More Than You Think

Here's one of the most frightening stats on our digital dependency to date: We now spend the equivalent of forty-four years of our lives staring at screens. According to the same 2020 survey, which was commissioned by the British company Vision Direct, those forty-four years break down into seventeen hours of screen time per day, with five hours spent on our laptops, four and a half hours on our smartphones, four and a half hours watching TV, and more than three hours spent on gaming devices. While your individual screen time may be less than this—other surveys have found the average American spends eleven hours staring at screens—your overall device time is still likely much more than you think: A separate survey found that 82 percent of all people believe their screen time is below national averages.

1. **You're dependent on your smartphone.** More than 70 percent of people who own a smartphone (which is more than 80 percent of all Americans) refuse to move more than five feet away from their devices. Over the past fifteen years, our phones have become our worlds, storing all our critical information and providing a means of instant communication we can't get anywhere else. Our phones are often our primary way to receive news; talk with friends, family, and colleagues; stay connected in the community; and function in most jobs, from medicine to manufacturing to retail to hospitality,

a reality that has only intensified during the coronavirus pandemic. Our phones also contain all our personal contacts, appointment calendars, music libraries, and photo albums. For many of us, the smartphone has taken the place of a traditional bank, wallet, camera, shopping cart, alarm clock, and basic wristwatch. In short, most people have become 100 percent dependent on their phones and can't imagine life without them—perhaps why one in three Americans would give up sex before relinquishing their devices.

2. **For many, dependency has led to digital addiction—an intentional move by many tech companies.** Approximately 90 percent of all Americans abuse, overuse, or misuse their personal devices, according to the Center for Internet and Technology Addiction. While this is an estimate and approximations of how many people actually have a digital problem vary, it's safe to say that many of us are suffering from some degree of technological addiction. How I define digital addiction is this: If your devices themselves—or the way you use social media and news apps on your devices—are interfering with your ability to do your job, manage your relationships, be present with family or friends, maintain a social life, or pursue hobbies or interests outside of the digital world, you may be addicted. You're also probably addicted to tech if it's affecting your physical health, mental health, sense of self-worth, or overall well-being.

While nobody thinks of our Facebook feeds or CNN apps the same way we do cocaine, the truth is that technology can be just as addictive as street drugs—and this problem can happen to anyone, no matter how old, successful, athletic, family-oriented, or sociable you are. That's because digital devices and media platforms work on the brain the same way that drugs do, triggering the same release of the feel-good neurotransmitter dopamine in the brain, and over time, causing emotional and mental withdrawal. Like alcohol and drugs, smartphones and digital media also act as social lubricants, emotional distractions, and ways to escape from reality. Like those who use drugs, many people also use their phones, check their social accounts, or surf the web when it's injudicious (like when their bosses are nearby) or dangerous (like when they're driving a car or walking down a busy street).

This addictive quality is by design: Digital media and our devices are designed to hook us and keep us hooked, minute after minute, hour after hour, and day after day. To quote *New York Times* op-ed columnist David Brooks, "Tech companies understand what causes dopamine surges in the brain, and they lace their products with 'hijacking techniques' that lure us in and create 'compulsion loops.'" These compulsion loops, specifically engineered by tech companies, cause us to keep repeating an activity because it gives us that dopamine burst— this is why we can't stop checking our social media feeds.

Tech companies hijack our attention by feeding us a constant stream of real-time news, notifications, and information, which in turn sparks fear of missing out, or FOMO—we can't ever look away because we're scared that we'll miss something. Social media in particular hooks us by encouraging us to do everything we can to get more likes, friends, and followers, giving us a fresh dopamine burst every time we get a hit, activating the same area of our brains as chocolate and money do. Social media and news apps feed us with shocking or frightful information, triggering a need to mitigate that fear by searching for more and more information. It doesn't stop there, either: Some digital platforms also hijack our appetites with the idea of scarcity, telling us that there are only so many minutes we can see a TikTok story, live Insta video, or online-dating match before it disappears, or that there are only so many of a product available for sale.

3. Whether you're addicted or not, technology is likely making you more anxious, depressed, stressed, lonely, and insecure. The research here is really clear: The rise of depression, anxiety, and suicide among teens and young adults over the past decade corresponds tick by tick with increasing rates of smartphone use among the same demographic. But you don't have to be in high school or college to experience the detriments: Studies show that smartphones, the internet, and social media can all increase depression, anxiety, loneliness, low self-esteem, and even self-harm in people of any age.

There are several reasons why tech triggers or worsens mental health issues. For one, social media causes us to continually compare ourselves to others, as we scroll through posts and pics of those who seem more beautiful, successful, popular, and smart than we are (even if those posts and pics are often curated, manipulated, or even paid for). This can drive up insecurity and cause a big self-esteem hit—studies show the more time you spend on social media, the more depressed and anxious you feel and the less satisfied you may be with your overall life.

While it may seem counterintuitive, the more time you spend being social online, the lonelier you're likely to be IRL (in real life), according to studies. That's partly due to the fact that spending time on social media means less time for hobbies, exercise, and socializing in person with friends and family, all of which are more rewarding than staring at screens, according to research. Although you might believe you have plenty of IRL relationships despite your device, surveys suggest otherwise: Six out of ten people say they spend less time with friends in the digital age, while 55 percent say social media has made their relationships "more superficial." This trend goes back as far as the 1960s, when TVs became ubiquitous in American households. Families stopped getting together with neighbors to socialize, and dance as a common social activity—from the twist to country line dancing—began fading out of our communities. The slow march toward screen-enabled social isolation has been going on for decades.

For the vast majority of my patients, I find that those who aren't strongly grounded to IRL activities like exercise, sports, family, their career, or the arts tend to lose their grip on reality alongside their sense of self-worth due to their relationship with social media. They become pawns in the digital media game, where depression, anxiety, isolation, and loneliness are the end result.

Social media isn't the only aspect to blame in the tech game, of course. Spending too much time on your phone reading news, surfing the web, or endlessly shopping can also trigger depression, anxiety, and isolation because it is distracting you from pursuing more meaningful activities. For these reasons, studies show that the more time people spend on their phones, regardless of how much of that time is on Facebook versus reading the *Wall Street Journal* app, the more stressed and burned out they tend to be.

Speaking of news, I have patients who argue that staying tethered to their news apps makes them more informed or smarter, not anxious, stressed, or depressed. I argue otherwise. Unless you're a day trader or politician, you don't need to get micromolecular news updates every hour: You can read the news once a day like world leaders used to do and still know everything important that's going on (in fact, you might know more, since you'll be reading more deeply rather than skimming over updates of old stories you've already seen). Otherwise, continually reading news exposes you to a cycle of negativity and fear—*if it bleeds, it leads*, as the saying in journalism goes— which only does double-time on your sympathetic nervous system (responsible for the body's fight-or-flight response), increasing your levels of cortisol, adrenaline, and anxiety.

Another problem with tech is that it allows us to be connected 24-7. Eighty-six percent of Americans say they check their email and social media accounts "constantly," which isn't making any of us any happier, according to research. Continual notifications of new emails and texts, as well as other alerts, also keep our sympathetic nervous system on high readiness, triggering a flood of stress hormones that can cause the brain's prefrontal cortex to malfunction, interfering with our ability to make decisions, practice good social behavior, and think about complex subjects.

4. **Technology may be worsening your brain fog, ADHD, memory loss, or poor attention span.** Recently, I've seen a ton of patients complaining of memory loss, poor concentration, or problems with brain fog. They tell me that they lose things constantly, can't remember things like names or tasks, feel jumbled, or just have a hard time focusing at work or on conversations with family or friends. Many worry they have early dementia or that a concussion incurred years ago is starting to manifest as permanent damage. Some ask for neurological testing, and if we order it for patients, 99 percent of the time they pass with flying colors.

It's not that these cognitive tests are easy—quite the opposite—but when people take them, they do so without their phones, laptops, smartwatches, and other personal devices. Without their tech to distract them, they have no problem focusing, remembering, and performing cognitive tasks. Why? Because when they take the test, they are present. Without constant bings, dings, and distractions, it turns out that our brains can work just fine.

This trend just isn't at my practice. In recent years, studies show Americans have experienced more brain fog, concentration issues, and attention deficit/hyperactivity disorder (ADHD)—

the latter of which has increased a whopping 43 percent among adults since the first iPhone appeared in 2007.

For me, the trend really hit home with a patient named Gail. A breast cancer survivor in her early seventies, Gail first came to see me because she was suffering from chronic inflammation and low-grade skin infections, which was an unfortunate result of the mastectomy she had had years before. At the same time, her health history revealed that she also had depression and ADHD. Gail was smart and successful, with a career as a theater director, but she told me that she couldn't function without Vyvanse and Adderall, both of which are commonly prescribed for ADHD. But even with the drugs, she was still having troubles with persistent brain fog and concentration.

While pharma companies claim these ADHD drugs aren't addictive, Gail, like many of my other patients, was hooked and had even developed a tolerance. I explained to her that I couldn't increase her dosage without risking serious side effects, like extreme jitteriness, heart palpitations, and a host of digestive issues, and that if she wanted to continue using them, she would have to go cold turkey for several weeks, then start again at a lower dose. Some of my other patients had had to do the same thing, either under my supervision or their psychiatrist's, which still often left them with withdrawal symptoms like exhaustion and increased brain fog and poor focus. For these reasons, I wanted to wean Gail off Vyvanse and Adderall entirely, but she was worried she'd be totally dysfunctional without them.

A year into working with me, after a couple of merry-go-rounds with her ADHD drugs, Gail, along with her husband, decided to take a two-month trip in a small sailboat they owned. Her husband was retired, Gail had her first free summer in years, they were both in their seventies, and sailing had always been one of the couple's bucket-list dreams. Out on the boat, though, there was usually no cell service or Wi-Fi, which meant there was no point in even bringing a computer or smartphone—and they had the ship's radio to call if they ever ran into trouble. Alone with her husband, who was an expert sailor, and without any work or students to vie for her attention, Gail said she didn't feel the need to focus or "be on," so she stopped taking her Vyvanse and Adderall.

Two months later, Gail walked into my office a different human being. Her depression and anxiety had faded, and she was finally able to focus on our conversations, along with her work, she added. While I had expected Gail to experience some attention difficulties due to withdrawal from her ADHD drugs, the opposite had occurred: She told me she no longer felt cognitively disabled, not because of the lack of any medication but because of the lack of any tech in her life: Without that ability to constantly check her email, news, social media accounts, the many listservs she was on, and all her other apps, she realized that she had far fewer problems focusing, recalling, paying attention, or being present.

Of course, very few people have the ability to take a few months to sail or completely unplug to this degree. But what both Gail's and Leah's stories show is that you may not be able to resolve your mental health issues, whether you have brain fog and ADHD or depression and anxiety, until you reset your relationship with tech.

Gail's story also highlights that people of any age can be addicted to their devices. I see so many older people who think their brain fog, poor attention, and memory loss are by-products of aging when their symptoms have nothing to do with cognitive decline and everything to do with digital dependency.

It's not just my opinion that tech triggers cognitive problems. Numerous studies show that smartphones cause memory loss, with one study finding that using a phone for as little as five minutes can lead to "significant memory impairment." In this last study, researchers in Greece asked participants to remember a computerized list of ten words they were shown once at three different intervals: before using their cellphones, immediately after using their cellphones for just five minutes, and another five minutes after the second measurement was taken, during which they didn't have access to their phones. People were able to recall the list of words the best before using their cellphones, not surprisingly, but the second best on the last interval, when more time had elapsed between seeing the words but also from using their phones.

While these studies may emphasize the extreme, our reliance on smartphones means we never have to flex our memory muscle, since we don't need to remember phone numbers, directions, appointments, addresses, or any other information we can now pull up online whenever we want. At the same time, our smartphones distract us from whatever we're doing in the present, interfering with our ability to learn new things and make memories. They also encourage multitasking, which can not only cause significant memory impairment, according to experts, but is also downright inefficient.

Your memory isn't the only thing at stake when you stare at screens all day: Your ability to focus and concentrate also gets dulled and begins to deteriorate. When you google, scroll, stream, click, or text—or do several at the same time—you never have to pay attention for longer than several seconds, and your brain gets used to switching from bite to bite to bite. Over time, your mind begins to require the same kind of stimulation to focus on anything, whether it's on or off a screen. This is one reason why the average American attention span has recently dropped by 30 percent, from twelve seconds to eight seconds. To put that into perspective, a goldfish can focus longer.

With our collectively crappy attention spans, it's not exactly surprising that rates of ADHD have soared. According to University of Wisconsin–Madison neuroscientist Richard Davidson, technology has created a "national attention deficit" that isn't unintentional: In his words, "We're all pawns in a grand experiment to be manipulated by digital stimuli to which no one has given explicit consent."

The deeper tech becomes ingrained in your life, the more you may be prone to attention disorders and impaired thinking. Studies show that people who didn't grow up using smartphones can concentrate better on complicated tasks and do more complex thinking, in part because their minds don't need to be distracted every second. This is also reflected in their moods, with people who are able to focus and immerse themselves in tasks often happier than those who can't do either very well, according to research.

Technology isn't just harming our cognitive abilities. It's also interfering with the structure and function of our brains, making them smaller, slower, and murkier, according to research. Studies show that technology use can actually shrink gray matter in the brain's frontal lobe, where all our high-level thinking and executive function occur, including planning, decision making, organizing, and impulse control. At the same time, staring at screens all day can damage the brain's white matter, which facilitates communication between different areas of the brain. Consuming too much tech also impairs how well you process information and perform tasks, according to research, while staring at your smartphone all day can create neurotransmitter imbalances that slow down cognitive function, also increasing the risk of depression, anxiety, and mental fatigue.

5. **Technology is seriously screwing with your sleep—and for reasons that go beyond blue light.** According to the CDC, inadequate sleep is a public health epidemic, as at least one out

of three Americans don't get enough sleep for general health (and this percentage is likely higher in actuality). Whether you're not sleeping long enough (less than seven hours per night) or you are but aren't getting enough deep sleep, being short on shut-eye can worsen or spark depression, anxiety, brain fog, and just about every other mood disorder possible.

If you know you struggle with sleep problems, you're ahead of the curve: Most people who are snooze-deficient aren't even aware that they're not getting enough sleep. Instead, they assume that the symptoms of poor sleep, which include low energy, increased appetite and cravings, irritability, brain fog, sadness, and an inability to concentrate, are just normal.

Lots of factors can cause poor sleep. But recently, I've seen more and more patients for whom technology is the primary driver behind their inadequate sleep quality or quantity. This isn't just because phones, computers, TV, tablets, and laptops emit blue light, which most people know by now can interfere with the body's production of melatonin, the hormone that makes us sleepy. When it comes to preventing sleep, blue-light interference is actually secondary to the issues caused by the stimulation that screens trigger. You can use all the blue-light filters and glasses you want, but if you're staring at a phone, computer, TV, tablet, or laptop right up until the time you go to bed, you're fueling the same cortisol rush and fight-or-flight overdrive we've discussed throughout this chapter. This means your body is in a state of hyperarousal, with no natural cues that it's bedtime, so it can't just turn off because you want it to. That's the equivalent of flying a plane at five hundred miles per hour and expecting it to stop on a dime because you want it to stop.

In other words, sleep isn't a mental decision you make but a physical state you have to enter. We need internal and external cues from both our body and our environment to be able to fall asleep, stay there, and spend enough time in deep sleep, the most restorative stage. Cues like the setting sun, dimmer lights, and less mental stimulation tell the brain's master clock, otherwise known as the suprachiasmatic nucleus (SCN), that it's time to lower our internal temperature, slow our heart rate, and increase melatonin production, all of which we need to fall asleep. Technology hijacks all these cues, making it next to impossible to get a healthy amount of sleep quality or quantity.

Screens aren't the only things to blame when it comes to the relationship between technology and poor sleep. Most people don't think of electric lighting as tech, but it absolutely is, developed by some very smart people to help make human existence easier. And while it does that, electric lighting also prevents the brain from getting the right cues that it's time for bed, as we stay bathed in a bright, artificial glow throughout the night. What's more, LED and fluorescent lighting are super-stimulating to the nervous system due to their constant flickering, which is imperceivable to the eye but super-irritating to the sensory system, like constantly tickling the brain with a feather.

Some patients tell me there's no way tech interferes with their sleep because they can fall asleep with their laptop open in bed or the TV on. Unfortunately, these may be just signs of how exhausted or sleep-deprived you might be, not necessarily indicators that tech isn't an issue for you. While many people have habituated themselves to watching a show on their laptop or television to "unwind" and get them into a mode for sleep, this is a habit, not a need—you don't actually *need* to watch the show to fall asleep. It's very similar to drinking a glass of wine before bed: The habit may appear to help you sleep, but in reality, wine or any type of alcohol will only steal from later sleep cycles. In the instance of watching TV before bed, you're stimulating your mind and disrupting natural sleep cues, which can interrupt your sleep cycles throughout the night.

Reboot Your Relationship with Technology

How can you change your relationship with technology when it's embedded in every aspect of your life? It's the same question all my patients ask. And while it may seem like a daunting proposition, it's possible to do. I know because I've done it and helped hundreds of other people do it, too.

Tech is a big part of my DNA as both a doctor and a member of the millennial generation. I don't suffer from chronic or severe mental health issues, but just like anyone else who stares at screens all day, tech still impacts my mood, making me anxious, irritable, scattered, inattentive, and even sometimes depressed. To me—and to anyone else reading this book who wants to have a State Change or just live optimally—that's not acceptable. At the same time, I know that I can't get rid of tech or even significantly reduce how long I stare at screens. So, I've developed a system to create a healthier relationship with tech that puts both you and me in the driver's seat without impacting our work or productivity, while also substantially lifting our mood. These adjustments, while simple, can help you have a major mood shift, too, resetting how technology influences your mental health.

1. **Set a one-hour daily time limit on all social media, total.** (**Yes, I said total.**) Most people spend hours on social media every day without even realizing how much time they're wasting. They check their apps in the morning, periodically throughout the afternoon, and then at night after work, and suddenly, they're averaging three hours per day staring at platforms known to make us anxious, depressed, insecure, and lonely. That's why I tell all my patients to set time limits on social media, especially since this is so easy to do. If you go into the "settings" feature of your smartphone, you can program a cumulative daily time limit for all social media apps—when you exceed it, your phone makes those apps inaccessible. While you can override the limit, I've found most patients don't, especially when they realize how much time they're

spending scrolling. What should your daily time limit be? I suggest spending no more than one hour total on all social media platforms per day. Any longer is a sizable percentage of your waking hours that will make it very difficult to treat or reverse any mental health issue.

If you're an influencer or work in social media, limiting social media may be difficult, since it's a big part of your work and how you communicate with clients or your community. But there's a difference between creating a focused post as part of your work and allowing yourself to scroll the Gram or Facebook for hours. Keep your scrolling hours to a minimum—no more than one hour per day—and home in on creating great content while you're "at work" on social.

2. **Set an overall limit for phone screen time.** Even with a time limit on social media, if you're like most Americans, you still spend hours every day on your phone, texting, emailing, surfing, shopping, playing games, and using other apps. That's why I recommend programming an overall limit on screen time, too, which you can do in your phone's "settings" feature. What's a good time limit? I suggest you start by learning the daily average of hours you spend on your phone, also available in the "settings" feature, and then cut it down by one-third—a good approximation of how much idle time (i.e., when you're doing nothing productive) that people spend on their phones. For example, if you currently average three hours screen time daily on your phone, set a total time limit of two hours. Use that extra hour to read, cook, take a bath, exercise, visit with friends, or do any other IRL experience that will ultimately be more satisfying or rewarding than scrolling and clicking.

3. **Avoid all screens one hour before bed.** How you spend your final minutes before bed has a huge impact on your sleep

quantity and quality. If you're like most people, you spend your final hours before bed stimulating your body and brain with TV, tablet, phone, laptop, video console, or computer, keeping yourself in a state of hyperarousal that interferes with the body's natural cues for sleep. Even if you use blue-light filters on all your devices, it's still critical to avoid screens for at least one hour before bed in order to reduce stimulation and allow your body the time it needs to calm down. I suggest setting an alarm on your phone to remind you to go tech-free one hour before bed and also programming your phone then to go into "do not disturb" mode, so that you're not tempted by buzzes, pings, or other notifications. At the same time, dim the lights and find another way to entertain yourself, since most people use tech to escape at night or avoid being alone with themselves. Personally, I've learned to love my alone time—and I have seen many patients realize the same thing. Instead of turning to tech, create a new nighttime ritual where you stretch, do yoga, read a book, prep your meals for the next day, take a bath, have sex, listen to relaxing music, paint your nails, or practice another form of self-care.

4. **Switch 25 percent of video calls to audio only.** These days, video calls are as common as the computers on which we host them, having almost entirely replaced regular audio-only calls since the onset of the COVID-19 crisis. Whether or not you've returned to an office, you're likely still dealing with Zoom, FaceTime, Skype, WhatsApp, and other video-chatting platforms. The only problem: Research shows that video calls are more exhausting than face-to-face meetings or audio-only calls, according to experts, since the brain has to work harder to try to interpret facial cues without being able to see hand gestures or other body language. If you're Zooming with more than one person, a split-screen or gallery view can also increase

fatigue, as you continually rivet your attention and likely have a more difficult time concentrating on what's being said. For these reasons, try to schedule old-fashioned, audio-only calls whenever a video chat isn't absolutely necessary.

5. **Marie Kondo your digital space and tidy up.** You may already know that having a messy home or office can lower your productivity level, focus, mental acuity, and even overall happiness. The same goes for having a messy digital space. If you're someone who keeps a dozen tabs open on your browser, has a cluttered desktop, or has 152 unread texts or emails, it's time to do a little cybercleaning. Close all tabs and programs on your laptop or desktop that you're not using and prevent apps like Spotify or Adobe from automatically launching every time you open your computer. Next, take some time to organize your desktop, grouping shared items or projects in named folders. On your phone, delete apps you don't use and clear out unread texts and emails. Yes, cleanup time should be counted in your daily allotment of screen time. By the way, I'm supremely guilty of having too many tabs open and letting my inbox get crazy. Every three months I do an inbox sweep of sometimes hundreds of unread emails, bringing the number down to fewer than ten. It's deeply satisfying.

6. **Set your devices to "do not disturb" during big projects or tasks.** When you're trying to concentrate on a big project or task, there's no need to be mindlessly checking your phone, too— doing so will only slow down your productivity and increase the time it takes to complete whatever you're doing. Setting your phone to "do not disturb" when you're working hard on another project, whether it's a work job on your computer or an endeavor in your home, will boost your focus and efficiency and help you finish the project or task in a fraction of the time.

7. **Put your phone away—really.** Most people never disconnect
from their phones no matter what they're doing or who they're
with. But when you keep your phone on and out at dinners,
movies, parties, and other social occasions, it signals to you
and everyone around you that you're willing to be distracted at
any minute. Not only is this rude, it's also highly disorganizing
for your brain: Studies show we don't fully focus on what we're
doing or enjoy outings as much when our phones are within
sight, even if they never ring, ping, or buzz. Other research
shows keeping your phone out at dinner makes you less happy,
while multitasking between screens and social events can
cause short-term memory loss and brain fog, exacerbating
the inability to be present and an overall dissatisfaction with
social activities.

Three High-Impact Ways to Overhaul Your Relationship with Tech

If you suspect technology is interfering with your mental health or you have anxiety, depression, brain fog, ADHD, isolation, or any other mood issue that's not getting better, you'll likely need to go further in upgrading your relationship with screens in order to get a meaningful impact. I recommend anyone with a mood disorder or who suspects technology is impairing their ability to feel optimal take the following three steps, which can help overhaul their relationship with tech. Again, you don't have to stop using your devices altogether, but you likely need to set several significant boundaries in order to reduce the constant stress and hyperstimulation tech is causing you. This may be the only way you'll be able to boost your focus, interpersonal relationships, sleep quality, and general happiness.

1. **Replace evening and weekend screen time with analog
   activities.** Screens entertain us and prevent us from ever
   having to be bored or uncomfortable, which isn't a good thing.
   Today, most people spend almost all their leisure time inhaling

technology and have absolutely no clue what to do when they don't have a screen to turn to. Take, for example, an interesting study conducted by Georgetown University computer science professor Cal Newport. When Newport asked 1,600 volunteers to do a monthlong "digital declutter" with him, he discovered that the most difficult aspect for many was that they had no idea what to do if they couldn't use social media, play video games, read online news, or stream anything. Instead, Newport encouraged them to find "high-value leisure activities" they enjoyed, like reading, writing, listening to music, making art, or spending more time with their children or families. Those who took his advice, he found, were rewarded with "a magic pill of sorts for curing the low-grade anxiety and existential aimlessness that define our culture of constant connection." In other words, those who replaced screen time with analog activities that they enjoyed became instantly happier.

I've seen the same thing in my patients. When they find an IRL activity they love to do, it shifts their entire world order: All of a sudden, they don't feel bored or uncomfortable without a screen, and they become less anxious and stressed and much more focused and present—and significantly happier. The trick, of course, is forcing yourself to find IRL or analog activities that you love. But just like you learned to brush your teeth and tie your shoes as a kid, you have to learn to create or find your own joy—it's a life skill. And when you do, you'll learn to take back something significant for yourself instead of allowing all your attention and time to be dominated by what others want to show or feed you.

Like Newport, I suggest finding high-quality activities that let you learn something new, challenge your skills or intellect, or allow you to be more present with yourself, your family, or your friends. The analog activities I now love to do at night after I put my kids to bed, instead of going back to staring at a screen, are to practice yoga, take a bath, or cook a meal. This last hobby I've only recently rediscovered after a period of relying on my husband to be the cook in the family, and now I find the process of cooking to be incredibly grounding and rewarding, whether I make a meal with friends or family or take the time to experiment with new recipes on my own. Some of my patients like to take long walks, read, paint, do creative writing, or even just listen to the radio. Whatever you like to do, I promise there is an analog activity that will bust your boredom and discomfort better than any screen and be your own magic pill for finding a State Change.

2. **Designate one screen-free day every week.** I want you to take one day every week where you don't stare at screens. This may sound frightening at first, but going screen-free for twenty-four hours can be one of the most rewarding things you ever do. You'll be more present and focused, and enjoy yourself, during this twenty-four-hour time period. For me, going screen-free on Saturdays actually makes me feel like I have a weekend rather than barreling through the workweek just to do more work over the weekend and/or play catch-up on social media, shopping, online news, and emails. Now, though, I use Saturdays to be present with my family and friends, and the time is always so much more memorable and enjoyable than before, when my Saturdays weren't screen-free. You can experience the same thing for yourself: By forcing yourself to get out of the house, find new activities, and get creative with your downtime, I promise the end result will be more memorable and enjoyable than whatever you can do while hanging around staring at your devices.

You don't need to have a family or a partner to play with in order to take a screen-free day—spending time with yourself or making plans with friends is a great way to go tech-free for twenty-four hours. But no matter what you choose to do or whom you choose to do it with, I recommend planning a few activities in advance so you have things to do and won't be tempted to fall back on tech. This doesn't have to take a lot of work, however. In my household, we typically do the same things every Saturday: I take the kids to the park, I cook with my husband, we read together as a family, we reconnect as a couple, we each work out while the other watches the children, and we socialize with other family members or friends.

Once you do a few screen-free days, you'll also find it easier to limit your tech consumption the rest of the week. It's like building a muscle: When you start to retrain your brain, you'll discover that you can do more without tech, not because you have to but because you're happier, more focused, and less anxious when you're not tethered to a device.

3. **Do a digital detox for at least one week.** As we talked about earlier in the chapter, social media, online news, and other forms of digital media are designed to trigger anxiety, anger, envy, and insecurity because that's what gets people to click, scroll, like, and buy. But when you're exposed to these feelings for hours a day, every day, week after week and year after year, it can add up to a continual state of anxiety, anger, envy, and insecurity. You may not even be aware these emotions are hijacking your mood, because fear-evoking and envy-driving forms of digital media are so normalized now, but that doesn't mean these negative feelings aren't there and aren't having a big effect on your mental health.

The only way to stop the cycle and take back control of your own emotions is to give up digital media altogether. Since this is impossible or implausible for many people, the second-best way to regain control of your emotional health is to do a digital-media detox for at least a week—and up to thirty days if you're suffering from anxiety, depression, brain fog, sleep problems, or self-worth issues. This means no social media, online news, video games, TV shows, or anything you can stream, scroll, or watch on a phone or computer. You can still use your phone to text, call, and email, and most people still need to use technology every day at work. But when you're not directly communicating with someone else or working, you shouldn't be staring at a screen if you want to do a proper digital detox.

I know cutting out digital media, even for one week, can be difficult, especially since many of us use it as an escape. But hiding out in social media, online news, surfing the web, or playing video games isn't going to make you feel any better—for all the reasons we've discussed, it's only going to make you feel worse. Remember that the goal of these changes around tech is to give your body, brain, and emotional mind the ability to go into a state of healing and repair.

Some of my patients initially balk at the idea of doing a digital detox. But I can't tell you how many of them finally agree, only to tell me how much calmer, peaceful, and even euphoric they feel after a few weeks without any screens. Most patients who struggle at first with the idea of doing a digital detox also end up continuing to do it for longer since they find going screen-free to be so pleasant.

If you're worried about feeling disconnected during your digital detox, here are few tips. First, buy an old-fashioned print newspaper or magazine and read it—you'll also remember more of what you read than what you would pick up from scrolling online. While print papers don't give minute-to-minute updates, you'll likely discover you don't actually need these micromolecular updates and that you understand more of what's really happening by reading long-form, investigative articles without them.

Second, remind yourself of what you're really missing on social media, which is usually nothing. Most posts are trivial updates like what your friends had for lunch, the thirtieth photo of their kid in one week, or their latest semi-informed opinion on some political or social controversy.

If the proposition of no social media still makes you feel uncomfortable, tell your friends and family in advance that you're going offline and use your digital detox time to call, text, or meet in person, all three of which are more impactful ways to connect with people than through social media.

When my patients stop using digital media for at least a week, they discover that what they've been consuming through social media and online news is usually nice-to-know or totally trivial stuff—it's never need-to-know or life-changing information. It's a similar reflexive habit to eating food just because it's in front of you: We've all grown accustomed to consuming digital media just because it's there, not because it is necessary, interesting, or even something that we want.

Finally, when you do a digital detox, remember that it's not a punishment. You're just gaining more time to be present, calmer, and content, more time to exercise and focus on your goals, more time to practice self-care, and more time to spend with family and friends. If there are people or issues that you feel tethered to only through social media and that you find yourself missing, use your newly discovered time to establish IRL contacts with those people or causes. Before you begin your digital detox, make a list of all the IRL activities you want to do, including friends you want to see, workouts you want to try, books you want to read, recipes you want to make, and hobbies you want to pursue. Use the time to discover a new sense of self and work toward the State Change we all have inside us.

CHAPTER EIGHT

Supplements to Change Your Energy and Flow

Most people fall into one of two categories when it comes to their thinking on supplements: Either you see them as overpriced hocus-pocus, or you've got drawers full, cabinets bursting, and shelves lined with hundreds of dollars' worth of supplements that you weren't sure ever worked, never finished, and now don't know what to do with. You may have also cycled through faith and disillusionment and are left somewhere in the middle, wondering what's next.

I sit in a third category: I believe supplements are potentially powerful tools that can improve physical and mental health. But in order for this to happen, it's really important that people take the right ones for them.

In my practice, I recommend pharmaceutical-grade nutraceutical supplements because I've seen over and over again how they help boost people's moods, focus, and energy in significant ways, sometimes even more effectively or sustainably than a prescription drug can. In some instances, a targeted supplement plan is all someone might need to transform their mindset from sad, anxious, foggy, or fatigued to balanced, calm, focused, or energized.

The thing about supplements, though—and a big reason why so many people think they're a waste of money—is that many brands don't work: They don't contain the active ingredients the label says they do, or they contain so little there's no way they can be effective. You also can't just pop supplements in whatever quantity or combination you want, whenever you want, and expect results. Supplements work when you take a scientific approach, using a high-quality product that's meant for you on a regular basis.

Despite how powerful supplements can be, I didn't learn about them in medical school. It wasn't until after I graduated and started training in functional medicine that I began to see just how potent certain naturally occurring nutrients can be in the body. This certainly doesn't contradict conventional medicine, since many of the world's oldest and most powerful drugs are made from plants. Even so, conventional medicine continues to overlook supplements as an effective treatment for many physical and mental health conditions, which is a big fail in my opinion. Many supplements are evidence-based, with research to show how they can help treat certain issues as effectively as prescription medications, with fewer or no side effects.

Today, I don't just prescribe supplements, I also take them. And if I don't take certain supplements every day, my mood suffers. I have a genetic variant of the MTHFR gene, along with more than two-thirds of Americans. Those with variants don't have a disease or genetic mutation—a variant is just a different DNA sequence from what's standard—but we can't fully absorb vitamin B_{12} and folate (also known as B_9) from food. Not getting enough B_{12} or folate can lead to physical ailments like weight gain and headaches, in addition to depression, anxiety, fatigue, irritability, brain fog, and other mood issues.

Addressing MTHFR variants and preventing the mood problems they can cause is easy: You can take methylated B_{12} and methylated folate on a daily basis, which I'll detail on page 199. Methylation, a process that occurs in the body to help repair DNA, allows those with MTHFR variants to absorb B_{12} and folate, which, for some, can significantly improve the physical and mental symptoms associated with low nutrient levels.

Before I began taking methylated B_{12} and folate, I would often be anxious for no reason and feel tired despite sleeping well, night after night. But soon after I did genetic testing and started supplementing eight years ago, my anxiety improved dramatically; not only that but my focus, energy, and emotional resiliency all improved as well. Today, I only feel tired and anxious when I forget to take my B supplements for a few days in a row, don't get enough sleep because of my kids, or have a fire going on at work, which we all know is part of life. This is empowering, since I now know that if I wake up in a funk or feel on edge, I can support myself in correcting the problem naturally with a healthy supplement that has zero downside.

Before we delve into the details, I want to be clear about what supplements can and can't do. A supplement alone is not going to cure major depression, post-traumatic stress disorder, schizophrenia, or another severe mental health condition. A supplement alone also can't undo the neuroinflammatory effects of a high-sugar diet, little to no exercise, irregular sleep, or too much time with tech. But for millions of people with depression, anxiety, brain fog, ADHD, or low energy, a high-quality supplement that's targeted, personalized, and used the right way can be game-changing, providing the specific boost you need to shift your mood.

That's what happened with Jennifer, who came to see me for migraines and weight gain. I started by giving the forty-eight-year-old mother of two a full hormone evaluation to assess her thyroid, adrenal, and sex hormones. Like a lot of moms I see, Jennifer was dealing with mild adrenal fatigue and a sluggish thyroid, and we started cleaning up her diet. We also worked on her sleep hygiene, since she was waking up in the middle of the night even though her kids were now sleeping a full ten hours, and to get back to sleep she needed options other than watching Netflix at 3 a.m. But then COVID-19 hit, and by summer of 2020, Jennifer didn't just have migraines, she also had acute anxiety, as she, like so many Americans, began to feel panicky about her health, livelihood, and the state of the world at large. Without any of her usual social outlets, and with her children and husband constantly at home, Jennifer began to feel jittery during the day and had trouble concentrating, as her sleep issues deteriorated from waking up at 3 a.m. to not being able to fall asleep at all.

I knew we needed to treat Jennifer's anxiety stat, since it was impacting her quality of life and changing how she saw others, the world around her, and, most critically, herself. Another doctor would have likely prescribed Jennifer an antidepressant or antianxiety drug, but I knew her mood issues were situational rather than the result of a chemical imbalance in her brain that we needed to correct. I also didn't want to put her on a psychiatric drug like Xanax or Valium, both of which can be addictive and potentially worsen mood issues over time due to the drugs' rebound effect.

In Jennifer's case, a single supplement was effective for calming her anxiety and improving her focus and sleep. While supplements work differently in everyone, the supplement that helped Jennifer get back to baseline was a blend of L-theanine—an amino acid that can produce relaxation—and GABA, or gamma-aminobutyric acid, a natural neurotransmitter that reduces anxiety and increases well-being. I prescribed this blend to Jennifer from a high-quality medical-grade brand, which she took every day, twice a day, morning and night. Two weeks later, her anxiety had nearly abated, even though the pandemic didn't end, and she didn't change anything else about her routine or habits. The supplement blend simply gave Jennifer's body and brain the support she needed to manage her stress and anxiety.

This was a huge win in my book. We had treated Jennifer's anxiety by using something gentle, safe, and nonaddictive, without significant side effects or tolerance risk. Her story reminds me how powerful supplements can be when used at the right time for the right person in the right way.

So where can you get started? I want to begin with the basics before we get fancy. Here, I'll detail four specific supplements I believe everyone can take every day, regardless of existing physical or mental health issues, all of which can help improve your mental resilience.

From there, I'll walk you through a targeted set of supplements you can add to help address symptoms like anxiety, stress, depression, poor focus, and low energy. This can help you personalize your supplement routine, taking only what you need and nothing extra.

But first, there are some things to know about supplements if you want them to work. If you've tried taking supplements in the past with little to no success, pay attention: What I'm about to share can help you finally unlock the power of plant-based medicine. That's because how you take supplements, including where you get them and how you combine them, can be just as important as which ones you take.

The Exact Science of Supplements: Twelve Things to Know to Find Something That Works

At the end of the day, there are thousands of supplements. But not all are created equal, more is definitely *not* better, and the "it can't hurt" approach is almost never the right one to take. If you want to see results, here's what you need to know.

1. **Most supplements don't work.** Most supplements sold in grocery stores, drugstores, and big-box retailers aren't effective. The supplement industry is poorly regulated by the FDA, which tests only 1 percent of the sixty-five thousand products available, and products often don't contain what they say they do in the amount listed on the label. A 2015 investigation, for example, found nearly 80 percent of supplements sold at GNC, Walmart, Walgreens, and Target didn't include the DNA from the plants listed on the label.

So what does work? At Parsley Health, we use only pharmaceutical-grade supplements that are sold primarily through licensed health practitioners like doctors, nutritionists, pharmacists, and certified acupuncturists. Pharmaceutical-grade supplements receive the kind of scrutiny that pharmaceutical drugs do, with third-party testing to make sure they contain 99 percent of the ingredients in the amount specified by the label. Pharmaceutical-grade supplements must also be absorbed by the body in no more forty-five minutes and can't contain any of the fillers, binders, or dyes that grocery-store supplements often have. Pharma-grade supplements usually cost more than grocery-store brands, but when your other option is buying something that likely doesn't contain what it says it does, the additional expense is worthwhile—the difference between getting what you want and throwing your money away.

While there are many amazing pharma-grade brands, the companies I've worked with for years and trust are Metagenics, Xymogen, Ortho Molecular Products, Thorne, Pure Encapsulations, and Gaia Professional (the professional line, not Gaia's direct-to-consumer brand). If you're unable to find these brands, or cost is an acute issue for you, I also like Jarrow and

Solgar, which are sold in many health food stores and tend to be less expensive but still have a good reputation for quality.

No matter which brand you choose, be sure to read the full ingredients list, not just the active or primary ingredients, before you buy. Some supplements, especially those that are lower in quality, contain added fillers, binders, or other ingredients, including soy, gluten, or dairy, that may be problematic for you or cause an allergic reaction.

Finally, the best form of a supplement, whether you choose a pill, tablet, powder, or liquid, is the one you're most likely to take on a daily basis. Don't opt for a powder, for example, if you won't be able to or can't mix it into water, juice, or a smoothie every day. The only exceptions are a few particular supplements—in Jennifer's case, her GABA and L-theanine blend—that should ideally be taken in liposomal form, meaning the nutrients are suspended in tiny fat particles, for optimal absorption.

2. **Supplements aren't drugs, so stop treating them like they are.** Despite how powerful supplements can be, most don't work as quickly or in the same ways prescription drugs do. You can't just pop an herb and expect it to chill you out in an hour like Xanax can. Compared to synthetic drugs, supplements work on a slower, deeper level. This can be a better way to treat mental health conditions, since a gentle improvement in mood is often more sustainable than a sudden jolt or suppression of symptoms. And while they may work more subtly, they still work and can change the way you feel, even if they require several days, weeks, or even months of daily use.

3. **More isn't always better.** Lots of people take everything but the kitchen sink when it comes to supplements, assuming that more is better—or that more certainly can't hurt. Using this strategy, they have no idea what's causing them to feel more

calm, positive, or energized . . . or terrible. On the other end of the spectrum, some people sprinkle a nutrient or herb into their morning oatmeal or afternoon smoothie, hoping to see results. With this approach, they never take enough consistently to get any effect—like taking a quarter of an antibiotic sporadically and expecting it to cure a sinus infection. Supplements, like drugs, have minimum necessary doses to be effective, and almost all need to be taken daily for several weeks before you'll see meaningful effects.

4. **Recognize the power of one.** The best way to truly tell whether a supplement is working for you is to isolate each individual ingredient at a time to evaluate its efficacy. With the exception of the Starter Kit on page 198, which consists of foundational nutrients, I don't suggest starting more than one supplement aimed at addressing energy, mood, or focus at a time. Instead, I recommend waiting at least three weeks before adding other nutrients, using the time to track and evaluate what each option does for your mood. With this approach, you know if something works without wasting money.

This reminds me of Janet, a fifty-five-year-old woman who came to see me after working with a big-name functional medicine doctor. This physician had prescribed her eight supplements, which she bought for a small fortune and started taking immediately after their first appointment together. When I saw her, she was still taking all eight; when I asked her if any had made her feel better, physically or mentally, she shrugged and said she had no idea. I suggested she stop taking everything so we could establish a baseline, then she could begin reintroducing one back at a time. She was surprised. *Really, stop them all?* She asked. I mentioned that some of the things she was taking were redundant, while others might not be targeting her primary concern, which was anxiety.

After she overcame her surprise, Janet stopped taking everything for two weeks. When she started to feel more anxious again, I recommended she restart one of the herbal blends she had been taking to see if that helped first. Her anxiety improved to where it had been before she stopped the supplements, which indicated the other products she used weren't making a big difference for her. From there, I added two foundational supplements for immunity, mood, and energy. The end result was that Janet went from taking eight products to only three, which worked better for her overall health than the boatload of supplements she'd been on before.

5. **Herbal blends can be optimal.** In the instance of some supplements recommended in this chapter, you may find products that contain more than one of the ingredients I suggest—and that's okay, especially if the additional ingredients are also listed in this chapter. While blended supplements may seem to contradict my "power of one" rule, you'll still start by taking only one supplement at time— in this case, it'll just be a blended supplement instead of a single-ingredient one. Sometimes, there's a benefit to blends, too. Whenever you see the same nutrients combined in high-quality products over and over again, there's often a good reason: Some nutrients are more effective when taken together, like certain adaptogenic herbs, for example, which we'll go over on page 204. But not all blends are created equal: Some companies try to pack too many nutrients into a single pill, diluting their potency, which is why it's critical to buy blends from high-quality brands only.

6. **There's a reason why this book didn't start with a supplements chapter.** If you want to have a State Change, you shouldn't begin by revamping your supplement regimen.

There's a reason this book started with information on how to self-assess your health, get the right diagnostic tests, eat to lower inflammation, exercise to shift your perspective, and stare less at screens: If you're not doing most or all of these things, popping a supplement is unlikely to move the needle for you from red to green. Supplements are more powerful when added to a foundation of better health.

7. **Use the three-week rule.** Most supplements aren't going to turn around your mental health in twenty-four hours. Like some psychiatric drugs, they can require weeks to take full effect. At the same time, not all supplements are effective in all people, even if you take a high-quality, pharma-grade brand daily. Since we all have unique medical conditions, genetics, diets, lifestyles, metabolisms, and rates of absorption, what works for your friend, spouse, trainer, or doctor may not work for you. I recommend taking a new supplement daily for at least three weeks before deciding whether it works for you. After three weeks, if you don't notice a difference in how you feel, stop taking it and try a different supplement. How to tell if a supplement is making a difference in your energy and mood? Complete the symptom index tracker on pages 32–39 before you begin a new supplement and again in three weeks, paying special attention to your score in the mental health section and noting which symptoms may have improved.

8. **Cheaper supplements aren't more cost-effective.** Supplements can be expensive, especially some of the pharma-grade brands I recommend, which may be double or triple the price of mainstream products. While it can be tempting to purchase less expensive brands, remember that many mainstream products don't contain the ingredient you need, which means you're basically throwing your money in the toilet. I also believe in

quality over quantity. I've had plenty of new patients spend hundreds of dollars every year to take a dozen grocery-store supplements that don't do anything for them. Instead, I tell them to use the same amount of money to purchase a few high-quality products shown to be pure and effective. If something doesn't work, we don't use it anymore and find an alternative that does alleviate symptoms. It's that simple.

9. **The best time of the day to take supplements is when you'll remember to do it.** Certain supplements, like those that boost energy or promote sleep, work better when taken in the morning or at night, respectively. But if you struggle to remember to take your supplements in the first place, don't worry as much about taking them at a certain time of day—just do so when it's easiest for you to make them part of your regular routine. For me, that's at night: I keep my supplements on my bathroom counter and take them right after I brush my teeth—they're a reflexive part of my bedtime routine. I also prefer to take supplements with a little food in my stomach, since some nutrients can cause nausea or acid reflux on an empty stomach. For others, though, taking supplements in the morning is easier, and some of my patients tell me that doing so gives them a mood boost during the day. Either approach can work—what matters more than time of day is that you're consistent every day. And don't worry: You can take supplements with coffee as long as it doesn't bother your stomach.

10. **Don't listen to just anyone when it comes to supplements, including your doctor.** Unfortunately, many primary care doctors, internists, ob-gyns, cardiologists, and other doctors who aren't trained in functional or plant-based medicine don't understand supplements or aren't aware of which ingredients can treat which conditions in certain dosing. This, in turn, has

led many people to consult the internet, social media, personal trainers, friends, or family for advice on supplements. But I want to caution strongly against this strategy: No one should be making medical decisions about their health and body based on what worked for someone else or which nutrient a celebrity is selling on Instagram. Remember that supplements are powerful *and* can be dangerous. At the very least, they cost money, and no one should throw their cash at a nutrient that may not work or might even worsen the condition they're trying to treat.

While many medical professionals may be just as clueless when it comes to supplements, I still recommend making an appointment with a healthcare practitioner before starting a new supplement regimen. If you can, find a functional-medicine doctor who understands supplements and how to use them to treat specific conditions. There's another bonus to seeing a holistic practitioner: You can work with this person to get the diagnostic tests detailed in Chapter Four. These tests can be beneficial before you start to take supplements, since they can show you whether you have a nutritional deficiency or underlying condition that might affect which nutrients you need.

11. **Don't play doctor with your dosing.** While I suggest a dose range for all the supplements recommended in this chapter, you should work with your doctor or other licensed practitioner to determine what's best for you. At the very least, adhere to the dose recommended by the product you use and never increase dosing above what's recommended on your own. Taking too much of certain supplements can cause toxic side effects and lead to hospitalization. Taking too little of a supplement, on the other hand, can be problematic, too, since the dose may not be enough to trigger any meaningful benefits. And if you start

something new and don't feel well, listen to your body, stop the supplement, and call your doctor.

12. **Get medical help, not a supplement, if you have a serious mental health disorder.** If you have clinical depression, anxiety, or another serious mental health disorder, the first step isn't a supplement: Be sure to get guidance from a licensed professional right away. Supplements can still benefit you, but aren't your first stop.

SUPPLEMENT STARTER KIT SNAPSHOT

- Methylated B_{12} and folate, 800 mcg–1,000 mcg daily
- Omega 3-fatty acids (EPA and DHA), 1,300 mg daily
- Vitamin D_3, 5,000 IU daily
- Probiotics (*Bifidobacteria* and *Lactobacillus* strains), daily

---

The Supplement Starter Kit:
Four Foundational Nutrients Everyone Should Take Every Day

No matter who you are, which physical or mental conditions you want to treat, or how healthy you think you eat, I believe most people can benefit from taking four supplements: vitamin D_3, fish-based omega-3 fatty acids, probiotics, and a combination of methylated B vitamins, B_{12}, and methylated folate. For reasons I'll detail in the following pages, most people are either deficient or low in these nutrients, all of which can have a profound impact on mood and mental health.

These four supplements make up what I call the Supplement Starter Kit— where you need to start to lower neuroinflammation, trigger healthy neurotransmitter production, and plug possible deficiencies or inadequacies so you can prep your body and brain to have a State Change. These supplements are also safe, widely available, and relatively inexpensive.

I recommend taking the Supplement Starter Kit daily for at least three weeks before you add other nutrients to your regimen. For some, the Starter Kit is all they might need to correct any mood or energy imbalances. But if you take the Starter Kit for three weeks and still feel anxious, depressed, negative, low energy, or like you can't focus or concentrate, you can personalize your supplement program to target these conditions, as I'll detail in the next section. First, though, here's why you need to start with these four supplements for improved energy, flow, and mood:

Methylated B_{12} and folate, 800 mcg to 1 mg (or 1,000 mcg) of each daily: B_{12} and folate are two of eight essential B vitamins the body needs daily to function properly. Because B vitamins are water-soluble, your body can't store them, meaning you have to consume them every day. But most people don't eat enough Bs, found naturally only in animal products. Eating too much sugar, caffeine, alcohol, and/or refined grains, like most Americans do, also depletes Bs, along with too much stress and some prescription medications like birth control pills. What's more if you have a variant of the MTHFR gene, like many Americans do, your body can't fully metabolize B_{12} and folate from food or supplements that contain unmethylated versions. For these reasons, many people have inadequate levels, and low B_{12} and folate are the two most common nutritional issues we see at Parsley.

Having low B_{12} or folate can be a big problem, since inadequate levels can cause depression, anxiety, brain fog, and fatigue, in some cases without any other contributing factor. According to research, being low in B_{12} or folate may also prevent prescription antidepressants from working effectively.

The solution, however, is easy: Take a combination of methylated B_{12} and methylated folate, which is different from 99 percent of the B vitamins sold on store shelves. Why methylated? Methylation is a biochemical process that helps the body repair DNA, lower inflammation, detoxify, and fight off factors that can lead to chronic diseases like cancer and dementia. Methylated supplements support the body's methylation process by making B_{12} and folate more bioavailable so you can fully use them. For those with MTHFR variants, methylated B_{12} and folate can be game-changing, improving anxiety and brain fog with a single supplement.

If you don't have a MTHFR variant or acute mood condition, you can still benefit by taking a methylated form of B_{12} and folate, as most people don't consume these nutrients in adequate quantities.

Marine omega-3 fatty acids, at least 1,300 mg per day (800 mg EPA, 500 mg DHA): Marine omega-3 fatty acids are imperative to healthy cognitive function and mood, but nearly no one is consuming enough of them in meaningful quantities. Ninety-five percent of all Americans don't get enough eicosapentaenoic acid (EPA) and docosahexaenoic acid (DHA), the two marine omega-3s found primarily in fatty seafood. As we know from earlier chapters, EPA and DHA lower neuroinflammation, increase serotonin uptake, improve and preserve cognitive function, and can even prevent and treat depression, anxiety, and other mood disorders. Marine omega-3s also balance our overconsumption of inflammatory omega-6s.

There's another type of omega-3 fat, alpha-linolenic acid (ALA), often called the "plant" omega-3 because it's found in soy, flax, nuts, avocadoes, and other legumes and veggies. While you're likely consuming enough ALA, this omega-3 isn't biologically active in the body until it's converted into EPA and DHA—and only 5 percent of ALA is turned into EPA, with an even smaller fraction capable of becoming DHA.

All these reasons make supplementing with EPA and DHA critical to mood. But to reap the benefits, you need to get an omega-3 supplement made from fish: Vegan EPA and DHA supplements formulated from algae aren't as bioavailable, meaning your body will have a difficult time absorbing and using them. If you suffer from acid reflux or experience a fishy aftertaste when taking marine omega-3s, store your supplement in the freezer and take it when frozen, which will allow the nutrients to break down more slowly in your stomach, preventing side effects.

Vitamin D_3, 5,000 IU daily: Ninety-four percent of all Americans don't get enough vitamin D, which comes from both the sun and food. If you live north of the 37th parallel, like the majority of Americans do, your skin can't manufacture enough D from the sun except during a few months in the summer—and even then, that's only if you don't wear sunscreen or a ton of clothing or have darker skin, all of which reduce absorption.

As for food, only a handful of items naturally contain vitamin D—fatty fish is the top source. While a few foods, like egg yolks, contain some D, the amount is so low that you'd have to consume nearly two dozen eggs a day to meet your daily requirement. What's more, if you have a health condition like obesity, Crohn's disease, celiac disease, or liver or kidney disease, you're much more likely to be deficient in D since your body can't absorb the nutrient as well.

Why worry about your daily D intake? Low vitamin D is strongly associated with the development of mood disorders, including minor and major depression, anxiety, sleep conditions, and ADHD. Being short on vitamin D increases neuro-inflammation, interferes with healthy blood sugar, and can sabotage immune function, all of which boost the risk of mental and cognitive problems. Low vitamin D can also worsen mood swings, fatigue, and chronic pain, in addition to hair loss, weight gain, and other physical symptoms.

Not all varieties of vitamin D work the same in the body, though: You should take vitamin D_3, the most bioavailable form of the nutrient. Also choose a D_3 supplement that contains vitamin K_2: Since D_3 helps the body absorb calcium, taking vitamin K_2 at the same time ensures your body deposits calcium in your bones, not your arteries, where it can cause blockages. I recommend taking a daily D_3 dose of 5,000 IU, which is higher than the recommended daily allowance of 600 IU for people under age seventy set by the Institute of Medicine (IOM) several years ago. Since the IOM made this recommendation, researchers have said the institute underestimated the daily recommended allowance by a factor of ten.

Probiotics with the *Bifidobacteria* and *Lactobacillus* strains, taken daily: You know from previous chapters that your gut harbors a diverse community of trillions of microorganisms known as your microbiome. This microscopic sphere has a huge influence on our mind and mood, so much so that the gut is often called the body's "second brain." The microbiome is responsible for producing approximately 95 percent of the body's serotonin and can help lower neuroinflammation and increase cognitive and emotional function when your gut is healthy. When it's not, however, you risk developing depression, anxiety, brain fog, ADHD, sleep disorders, and overall mood dysregulation.

Unfortunately, most people don't have a healthy microbiome. Eating a standard diet rich in sugar, refined grains, vegetable oils, and food chemicals kills good gut bacteria, as do many prescription and over-the-counter drugs, outdoor and indoor air pollution, stress, and a sedentary lifestyle. For these reasons, everyone should consume more probiotics—healthy bacteria found in food and supplements. Research shows boosting probiotic intake can help prevent and treat mood disorders, while brain scans have found that people who consume high quantities of good bacteria have healthier cognitive regions associated with mood. Probiotics are so paramount to mood that researchers use the term *psychobiotics* to describe the mind-boosting effect healthy bacteria can have on psychiatric issues.

Some cultured dairy and fermented foods, like yogurt, kefir, kimchi, and sauerkraut, contain probiotics, but you need to be careful: Not all cultured dairy contains live probiotics, and heating or pasteurizing products like sauerkraut and kimchi will kill off the good stuff. What's more, some probiotic foods, like yogurt and kombucha, can be high in sugar, which undoes the advantages these products can have. It can also be difficult to get enough probiotics through food, especially if you're not consuming these items on a daily basis.

There are dozens of different strains of probiotics, and not all have been shown to improve mental health. In general, the strains research supports for mood and mental health are from the *Lactobacillus* and *Bifidobacterium* genus, particularly: *Lactobacillus (L.) rhamnosus, Lactobacillus casei, Lactobacillus helveticus, Lactobacillus plantarum, Lactobacillus acidophilus, Bifidobacterium bifidum, Bifidobacterium breve,* and *Bifidobacterium infantis.* To be sure you're consuming enough of these strains—and ones that are actually alive and effective—it pays to take a high-quality supplement.

That said, not all probiotic brands include live strains in the quantity they say they do on the label. While it doesn't matter if you choose a refrigerated version—freeze-dried strains can be stored at room temperature—make sure what you buy is formulated by a trusted manufacturer. I like our Parsley Health probiotic, which is made by Ortho Molecular, one of my top recommended companies. The MegaSporeBiotic, made by Megabiome Labs, and probiotics from Klaire Labs are also high quality.

Finally, I don't recommend a certain dosage of probiotics, because there's no evidence of any ideal number of colony-forming units (CFUs) for optimal physical or mental health. Instead of dosage, focus on getting a high-quality brand, which will help ensure you're receiving and have the best chance of absorbing healthy bacteria.

Using Supplements to Target Specific Mood Issues

Taking the Supplement Starter Kit daily for three weeks will give your body a leg up and help you support a healthy mood response. It's designed to get your body into a state of healing and help lower inflammation, but it's not a cure-all. After you begin the Starter Kit, you can add on additional supplements—one at a time, every three weeks—to address specific mood issues. To help you determine which supplement might be best for you, I've created three different categories, which target specific mental health symptoms:

- **Calm** to help treat anxiety and chronic stress
- **Mood Boost** to help treat depression, sadness, or persistent negative outlook
- **Energy and Focus** to help treat low energy, brain fog, and difficulty concentrating

Not sure where to start? I get it: You're human, which means you have a complex set of emotions that don't always fit neatly into boxes, codes, or categories. But getting clear on your symptoms can help get clear your goals. Ask yourself: *Of the three categories, which best describes the state of being I want to achieve? Which category targets the feelings I experience the most often?* This self-evaluation can not only help you choose a supplement but can also provide clarity on which issue impacts your life the most.

Why not supplement across categories? While you may be able to add from different categories after several weeks, you shouldn't mix and match right out of the gate. That's because what may work to calm you down could also potentially lower your energy if you're dealing with persistent fatigue. On the other hand, what might hone your focus could also increase your anxiety if that's your overriding concern. By focusing on one issue at a time, you'll be able to steadily reveal which products are best for you.

ALL ABOUT ADAPTOGENS: THE NEWEST BUZZWORD IN WELLNESS HAS MEDICAL CRED WHEN USED PROPERLY

Adaptogenic herbs, also called adaptogens, are plants that help the body adapt to stress. They can lower the amount of tension we feel and the toll it takes physically and mentally on our bodies and brains. Adaptogens have been used for thousands of years in Chinese medicine and other traditional medical practices worldwide. In the past several years, they've also become popular in mainstream Western markets, available in supplements and even functional foods and drinks that claim to help lower stress and promote calm.

Buzz aside, adaptogens have lots of research to show they can help mitigate anxiety and other mood disorders. I like them because they work with the body rather than working against it, to reduce stress and help people feel a greater sense of balance. In my practice, I recommend well-researched adaptogens like ashwagandha and schisandra for anxiety, along with ginseng and *Rhodiola rosea* for low energy. However, there are dozens of other adaptogens that may also be beneficial if your functional or holistic practitioner recommends something different. Just don't rely on functional foods and drinks that contain adaptogens—the dosage in these foods is usually insufficient and the quality too low to be effective.

Supplements for Calm

This category may be the most helpful, since most people suffer from some sort of anxiety or chronic stress. As you may remember from Chapter One, the ICD diagnostic code for anxiety is the most common one we see at Parsley Health. If you're experiencing chronic stress or anxiety, you're not alone. Taking a targeted supplement daily can help treat or even reverse the condition. Here are my top recommendations:

- **Ashwagandha, Schisandra, or a blend, with 200–400 mg ashwagandha and/or 100–200 mg Schisandra per day:** If your most troubling symptom is feeling on edge during the day, I would suggest taking ashwagandha, schisandra, or a blend that combines both. Ashwagandha has been used in Ayurvedic medicine for centuries to counter stress and increase feelings of happiness, while Schisandra is a fruit extract popular with Chinese medicine practitioners to treat a host of disorders, including anxiety. In my practice, patients who take ashwagandha, schisandra, or a blend of both tell me they are able to sustain a more energized calm during the day. If you find a high-quality product that blends both, start there, since these two adaptogens can work together to have an even more powerful impact. Ideally, you'll want to take this blend in both the morning and the evening for best results.

- **Magnesium glycinate or magnesium threonate, with 200–400 mg glycinate or 1 gm threonate per day:** If you have trouble relaxing at night or can't fall asleep because you're stressed or overstimulated, magnesium can be hugely helpful.

  As we covered on pages 140–41, magnesium is essential to three hundred different biochemical reactions in the body, including many that support our mind and mood, but at least half of all Americans don't consume enough of the mineral. Research shows that magnesium has a strong calming effect, so much so that I think of it as nature's Xanax. But to benefit from magnesium's chill-out potential, you have to get the right formulation. I suggest taking formulations with either magnesium glycinate or magnesium threonate, which are best absorbed by the body and won't cause digestive issues. Beware: A lot of the magnesium supplements on the market contain magnesium oxide or citrate, which isn't well-absorbed and is better used as a laxative.

- **GABA and L-theanine blend, with 600–800 mg GABA and 100–200 mg L-theanine per day:** Gamma-aminobutyric acid

(GABA) is a calming neurotransmitter produced by the brain also available in supplemental form. People who are constantly stressed often don't have enough GABA, since the body's fight-or-flight response drains the neurotransmitter. L-theanine is an amino acid found in green tea that's been shown to reduce stress and anxiety and also helps the body produce more GABA. I like to prescribe these two together to my patients who feel constantly overwhelmed or stressed. In this instance, if you can find both nutrients in liposomal form, which means the ingredients are suspended in fat-like particles, it will help your body better absorb them.

- **Phosphatidylserine (PS), with 200 mg per day:** Phosphatidylserine (PS) is a fatty substance produced by the body that helps you protect your brain cells. Plants also make PS, which is where the supplemental form of the nutrient comes from. Studies show PS helps regulate the stress hormone cortisol and can help obviate the kind of overnight cortisol response that wakes people up at two or three in the morning in a cold sweat. If anxiety is preventing you from sleeping through the night, start your additional supplement regimen by taking PS before bed.

Supplements for Boosting Mood

If depression, sadness, or negativity is disrupting your ability to experience joy, a mood boost supplement can help improve your outlook. If you're already taking an antidepressant, check with your prescribing doctor for potential interactions before adding any of these supplements. What's more, if you're already on a prescription antidepressant, these nutrients may not be hugely additive—the following recommendations are primarily for those looking for support for mild depression. Finally, none of the following supplements is intended to replace a prescription drug.

- **St. John's wort, with 300 mg per day:** St. John's wort may be the most popular and buzzed-about supplement on this list, touted for years as a natural antidote for depression. While research shows the flowering shrub can help effectively treat depressive symptoms, I've found the supplement's impact is binary: It either works really well or doesn't have much of an effect. If you've tried taking St. John's wort in the past and didn't see benefits, I'd suggest taking a high-quality brand daily for at least three weeks to make sure purity or consistency wasn't why it didn't work. If you don't notice a difference, try another nutrient in this category. But if it helps you feel more positive or, as I've found with many patients, helps you start to climb out of your funk, keep taking it.

- **5-hydroxytryptophan (5-HTP), with 100 mg per day:** 5-hydroxytryptophan (5-HTP) is a naturally occurring amino acid that helps the body make serotonin, which prescription antidepressant drugs like Zoloft and Prozac also do. Some studies have even found that 5-HTP can work as effectively as antidepressants, but with fewer side effects. If you suffer from mild depression, try supplementing with 5-HTP on a daily basis. If you're already on an antidepressant, this one may not be the best pick for you; speak to your doctor before trying it.

- **S-Adenosylmethionine (SAMe), with 200 mg per day:** SAMe is a chemical that aids in the body's methylation process. When taken with methylated B_{12} and folate as part of your Supplement Starter Kit (see page 198), SAMe can help regulate and increase production of dopamine, serotonin, and norepinephrine, all which help stabilize mood. In Europe, SAMe is available as a prescription drug and used to help treat depression; the nutrient has also been shown to increase the efficacy of antidepressant drugs. SAMe is a great addition to the Starter Kit if you feel better with these foundational supplements but want a bit more of a mood boost.

Supplements for Energy and Focus

This category can help you treat low energy, chronic fatigue, poor focus, brain fog, and support those with ADD/ADHD. But before you start popping a supplement for energy issues, you need to make sure you're sleeping long enough and well enough—if you're short on either sleep quantity or quality, an energizing supplement is unlikely to have any impact. Similarly, fatigue and brain fog are common symptoms of many underlying issues, including thyroid problems and nutritional deficiencies, so it's important to rule these out with the diagnostic testing outlined in Chapter Four.

I have plenty of patients who don't have sleep issues or underlying conditions but who do have low energy, fatigue, poor focus, brain fog, or attention difficulties. For these patients, the right supplement can make all the difference in how they feel, giving them a natural, nonaddictive boost. For best results, I recommend taking supplements for energy or focus first thing in the morning.

- *Rhodiola rosea,* **with 100–200 mg per day:** Of all the energizing supplements, I think *Rhodiola rosea* provides the most stabilizing increase in energy in a way to which most people respond well. If you have a mood issue like depression that's also depleting your energy, start with *Rhodiola rosea*: Research shows the herb can reduce symptoms of depression while also improving fatigue—in some instances, after just one week. *Rhodiola rosea* is also an adaptogen, so it can help you manage stress. The herb may also increase cognitive function, with some studies showing it improves mental performance by as much as 20 percent.

- **Panax ginseng and/or eleuthero, with 100–300 mg Panax and/or 100–200 mg eleuthero per day:** These two adaptogens work similarly to boost energy and focus in the body and brain. Panax, also known as Korean ginseng, contains active ginseng, while eleuthero, which used to be called Siberian ginseng, doesn't (why they changed the name). Panax is stronger and more expensive than eleuthero, with studies showing the former can effectively mitigate mental and physical fatigue while improving cognitive function. While the research on eleuthero isn't as strong, in part because it's not a stimulant like Panax, several studies have found supplementing with the adaptogen can increase cognitive performance. I find taking a blend of both can provide an energy boost similar to caffeine, without the dehydrating effect. If you're using coffee, energy drinks, or diet soda to get through the day, taking Panax ginseng with eleuthero can help reduce your dependency on these items while providing a more sustained source of energy that can last throughout the day.

- **Pyridoxal 5-phosphate (P5P), with 10–30 mg per day:** Persistent stress, whether it's psychological or physical, can deplete the body's stores of B_6, also known as pyridoxine, one of the eight essential B vitamins. B_6 is necessary to make many neurotransmitters responsible for balanced mood, along with the protein hemoglobin that carries oxygen in blood throughout the body. If you're facing chronic stress, you may want to take pyridoxal 5-phosphate (P5P), which is the bioavailable form of B_6, in addition to your other methylated B vitamins.

Supplements can be a power tool in your toolkit to help you have a State Change. For many of us, taking dietary supplements on a daily basis can fill out the nutritional gaps we have by providing critical nutrients—like B vitamins, marine omega-3s, vitamin D, and probiotics—that are essential to physical and mental health but often missing from our everyday diets. In addition, using certain supplements to target specific mood issues can help us manage symptoms in a more natural, gentle, and sustainable way than prescription psychiatric drugs. This is not to say you shouldn't take psychiatric drugs if you need them or are prescribed them; pyschotropic drugs are powerful, effective, and oftentimes lifesaving. But for many people, supplements can also be powerful and effective and can be part of any multipronged plan to elevate your baseline mental state.

CHAPTER NINE

The New Frontiers: Psychedelics, Meditation, and Energy Healing

Summer of 2020. The middle of a global pandemic. I was lying on a mat on the floor of a studio apartment on the Upper East Side of Manhattan, surrounded by gongs, tapestries, and tribal masks of unknown provenance. I'd just said a small prayer to the "little people," thanking them for their work and asking them to take me where I'd never been before.

This was not an everyday experience. Quite the opposite: I was there with a professional guide to try psychedelic drugs for the very first time—more specifically, the drug known as psilocybin, a hallucinogenic compound found in "magic mushrooms" that's been heralded for helping cure anxiety, depression, addiction, eating disorders, and other mood conditions. My reason had nothing to do with getting high and everything to do with trying to shift my mental outlook, which I'd heard from a number of colleagues, friends, and patients is possible when you agree to meet the "little people," a friendly moniker for magic mushrooms.

Still, the experiment went against nearly everything in my DNA. Like many Americans, I grew up believing that alcohol was normal, and that any other drug was taboo, if not a fast track for life destruction. In high school and college, I never experimented with recreational drugs other than smoking a little bit of marijuana, which I didn't really enjoy. Quite frankly, in my younger years I'd always been pretty afraid of drugs, and as I got older my priority has been my physical health and well-being, so anything that seems potentially toxic I've chosen to stay away from.

But over the last few years, my view of psychedelic drugs—a category of hallucinogenic substances that includes magic mushrooms, MDMA, peyote, ayahuasca, LSD, and ketamine—had changed. Today, I've joined many of my colleagues, including medical researchers and doctors, in believing that psychedelics like psilocybin are a promising new frontier in mental health, capable of treating or reversing mood disorders in a way psychiatric drugs have never been able to do. I've seen many patients turn around serious mental health issues in a matter of months by combining psychedelics with targeted therapy.

By the summer of 2020, I'd decided I had to experience what so many others before me had already tried. I didn't have any significant anxiety or depression, but I was aware of how my ego could get in my own way, how my sense of self was often tied to my achievements, and how my sense of reality could be rigid— meaning I used my conscious brain to constantly interpret and analyze rather than simply observing or letting things happen to me. I felt I needed to experience the mindset shift people kept telling me about, to understand how psychedelics can indelibly alter your understanding of consciousness.

That's how I found myself on the Upper East Side, spending a quiet summer Friday afternoon with a professional "trip sitter," watching as he broke up the psilocybin into applesauce for me to eat. I spooned it into my mouth, noting that it didn't taste any different from regular applesauce. Immediately afterward, I tried to relax, as I waited for things to begin. I had no idea what to expect, and what happened next was nothing like I'd imagined.

About twenty minutes later, a kaleidoscope of colors emerged out of the ceiling and from the walls around me. I reached my hand up to wave my fingers through the rainbow prism. Soon after, everything felt benevolent, and I found myself laughing out loud uncontrollably, as random thoughts floated into my mind, which I immediately deemed hysterical. This was what my guide told me is called the hinterlands—when your visuals begin to shape-shift and you start to walk from the conscious reality you think you know into one that isn't familiar at all.

Many people say taking larger doses of psilocybin can cause them to experience a phenomenon known as "ego death," where they no longer feel confined by their own identity. This occurs when the drug triggers a radical kind of uncoupling of who you are from who you think you are, which is exactly what happened to me. On psilocybin, I no longer felt attached to the things I'd used for years to define myself: my job as a doctor, my background from Baltimore, the education I'd received at various schools and universities, my body and how I looked physically, and how I thought others around me viewed me. Instead, I felt a kind of pure consciousness, as though I was simply floating, alive and selfless in the universe.

At times, this was a frightening feeling, and I was acutely aware of wanting to get back to a sense of self I could recognize. But other times, I felt like I was deeply aligning with what was important in life. Suddenly, it didn't matter what I did for a living, how much money I made, what I looked like, where I had gone to school, or any of the other external markers we use to define ourselves: The only important things were my children, my husband, the other people I loved, and the impact for good I could have through my work. This is what I wanted to return to while traveling through my psilocybin trip—not my title, accomplishments, bank account, physical body, or other external parameters I and so many other people use to define and measure ourselves.

This new sense of self and a deeper connection with the humans I love have lasted with me to this day. Afterward, I felt calmer and more healthfully detached from the day-to-day of my usual grind. I was acutely aware on both a physical and experiential level (rather than an intellectual one) of how my essence and identity weren't connected to the things I'd spent most of my life worrying about—my work, finances, home, education, etc.—which bestowed on me a sense of confidence and freedom. After my trip, I was able to see that who I am is eternal, untethered to these material or subjective markers. During my experience on psylocibin, I had moments of deep fear that I would stay in that state of unconsciousness forever, unable to return to my family and the life I knew, such that I formed an even deeper and more lasting appreciation for everything I have as I returned through the hinterlands and back to my normal state of consciousness.

More than a year later, I continue to thank the little people for reminding me that how we treat others is all that really matters. While I've known this intellectually for years, my experience with psilocybin showed me how to be less attached to the daily drama—not only while I experienced the trip but also ever since. I've still tried magic mushrooms only once; there is nothing addictive about them, and so far I haven't felt any urge to go back. But the one trip helped shift my sense of reality in a way that comes back to me sometimes during my day-to-day, similar to how traveling to a foreign country for an extended period of time can imbue your sense of self with a different dimension for years after the trip.

I'm sharing my story because I think it's important to strip the stigma that psychedelics have, for reasons I'll detail later in this chapter. I admit that I'm a novice in this area and that there are experts like acclaimed author Michael Pollan, biohacker Tim Ferris, and the many scientists and physicians leading research in the field who have much more to say on this topic than I do. However, I want to show you just how powerful these drugs can be, not just for doctors like me who are interested in understanding how they work in an academic way but for patients with serious mental health issues who can potentially end years of depression, anxiety, or other types of emotional anguish by experiencing a new sense of self or state of consciousness. Studies show that psychedelics can cure some people of mood disorders in just weeks or months, even after years of prescription antidepressants, talk therapy, or other conventional treatments have failed. One study from Johns Hopkins University's Center for Psychedelic & Consciousness Research, for example, found that a combination of psilocybin and therapy cured half of its participants with major depressive disorder in just one month's time, while the other half showed significant improvement in their symptoms.

I want to be clear from the start: There's nothing recreational about using psilocybin or other psychedelics for mental health reasons. The kind of psychedelics used for therapeutic purposes are different in dosing and purity than what you would find on college campuses or in clubs. What's more, for these drugs to be effective, they need to be used with what's known as integration therapy, which combines psychedelic treatment with professional therapy to help patients make sense of their "trip" so they can integrate the experience into their everyday lives. Integration therapy requires patients to meet with a licensed therapist trained in the technique and do the work to determine how they can harness the power of their psychedelic experience to get past mental or emotional blocks or redirect their treatment. Without integration therapy, if you take them recreationally or in an effort to self-medicate, psychedelics may not do anything for your mind or mood—on the contrary, recreational drug use or self-medication may exacerbate mental health issues.

When they're used appropriately for therapeutic purposes, I believe psychedelic drugs are one of the most exciting new approaches in mental health treatment. But these drugs aren't the only new frontier for the mind and mood. There are a number of other unconventional or forward-thinking healing practices that can help support your mental health, which is what this chapter is all about.

Research has shown us there are dozens of different ways to achieve flow state and transform mental health, many of which are more effective than therapy or medication, as we've covered in previous chapters. But if you want to do everything possible to achieve a State Change, it helps to put everything on the table, including those practices that, at first glance, may seem woo-woo or make you uncomfortable. Sometimes, going outside the box, challenging the norm, or challenging *your* norm is all that's needed to upgrade your mindset from "meh" to amazing.

In short, if a therapy exists that can help you transform your mood, even in the smallest way, I want you to know about it. There are three new frontiers for mental health that I believe everyone should be aware of, if not consider on a daily or regular basis: meditation, psychedelics, and energy work. We'll cover all three in detail here.

New Frontier #1: Meditation

Meditation isn't exactly a new modality, as it's been practiced for thousands of years. But it is a new frontier when it comes to conventional medicine and mental health treatment. When was the last time you heard of a psychiatrist prescribing daily meditation alongside Zoloft or Wellbutrin? It's a rare occurrence, even though meditation is the most powerful drug we have to disrupt our thoughts and how we think them.

That may sound radical, but MRI scans show that regular meditation changes both the structure and function of the brain, thickening critical areas like the hippocampus, which helps improve focus, attention, and emotional control, while shrinking the amygdala, the area of the brain responsible for initiating fear, aggression, anxiety, and stress. Studies also show meditation alters neural circuitry that makes people more compassionate while reducing activity in the brain's default mode network (DMN), which is responsible for mind-wandering.

There's something else that regular meditation does, too: It fills the ruts in the road of your mind, forcing your thoughts to have to find new routes. Let me explain why that's so critical to your mood and mental health.

According to neuroscientists, 90 percent of all thoughts are repetitive, meaning we think the same thing over and over again. Eighty percent of these repetitive thoughts are negative ones. You don't consciously choose what you think about—you just knee-jerk think, repeat, think, and repeat. This is kind of like using the same weight machines in the gym every day, allowing certain muscles to get really strong and good at accomplishing one specific movement while everything else atrophies. Thinking the same things over and over again just lets your brain get better at coming up with the same thoughts and conveying them quickly. In short, you create mental ruts for the same thoughts, and your brain rolls through these ruts over and over again because you've trained it to do so.

But the great thing about the brain is that it's wonderfully plastic, meaning it can change and actually rewire itself. If you want to rewire your automatic thoughts and change how you think, the most effective tool you have is meditation, which can thicken key areas of your brain, literally repaving the mental ruts in your mind. This forces your thoughts to find new pathways, which can effectively cut off long-standing anxieties, fears, insecurities, and destructive attachments. By meditating daily, even for only a few minutes per day, you can reprogram your thoughts and begin to feel and live differently, simply because you're no longer experiencing the same thoughts and reactions over and over again.

For all these reasons, meditation has been shown to be a successful treatment for depression, as effective as antidepressants in some instances, along with helping to reverse anxiety and mitigate stress. Studies also show that a regular practice can increase focus, learning, memory, and attention span. In addition, meditation lowers blood pressure and blood sugar, boosts sleep and immune function, and can help treat the symptoms of many illnesses, including cancer, chronic pain, and heart disease. If you've resisted the idea of meditation in the past, think of it this way: Meditation retrains your brain to have something I like to call the One-Second Superpower, the ability to take as little as one second of mental space (and up to a few minutes) between an internal emotion and an external reaction. This One-Second Superpower allows you to have a choice about how you want to interact with the world around you and whether you show more calm, clarity, and agency in your emotional responses.

When my husband makes a comment that really pisses me off or something goes haywire at work, for example, this One-Second Superpower helps me take a beat before flying off the handle or overreacting, allowing me to gather the poise, strength, and clarity to choose how to best react. This ability to choose your reaction can foster healthier relationships, both professionally and personally, and even prevent possibly dangerous behavior, like reacting with violence, substance abuse, or other potentially damaging habits.

How to Meditate the "Right" Way

What so many of my patients don't realize about meditation is that you don't have to be a monk to benefit. Quite the opposite: Studies show that as little as five minutes of meditation per day can cut stress. Do ten minutes per day, and you can overturn repetitive, negative thoughts while improving your cognitive function, memory, and creativity.

If you've tried meditation and found it too difficult or simply believe there's no way you can sit quietly with your eyes closed while concentrating on nothing, I'm going to let you in a big secret: The greatest mistake most people make is thinking they have to be instantly and totally Zen when meditating or they're somehow not doing it "right." This just isn't true. Your mind can wander, and it's okay if you don't feel serene. You don't even have to sit with your eyes closed: You can stand or sit with your eyes open. As long as you try to keep coming back to the present by focusing on your breath, a mantra (a word or phrase you repeat over and over), or something in your immediate environment that you can focus your eyes on, you'll disrupt your automatic negative thoughts.

Even though I've practiced meditation for years, my mind still wanders and gets distracted. Instead of letting myself get upset by it or throwing in the towel, I've learned that working through these moments can make them some of the most transformative. By refocusing on the present moment over and over again, I'm essentially building the muscle in my brain to experience presence. I know that when I bring my attention back to my breath and simply observe my thoughts rather than attaching myself to them, I'm filling those ruts in the road of my mind that automatic thoughts can create. When I do this regularly by working through distracting thoughts in meditation, I force my mind to travel new roads, which can lead to new mental, emotional, and creative revelations.

While some say you can meditate while exercising or otherwise moving your body—walking, for example, or doing the dishes, or even navigating your commute—I believe true meditation requires stillness in the body in order to facilitate stillness in the mind. Otherwise, it's all too easy to let motion distract you from mindfulness, as you sustain that frenetic energy that so many of us, me included, use to prevent experiencing the present or unpleasant thoughts or emotions.

Meditating while doing some form of cardio that relies on repetitive movement, like running, biking, or walking, may be popular right now, but I believe the repetitive nature of these types of workouts just keeps your mind locked on its repetitive thought cycle. I also don't recommend using yoga as a primary path for meditation. While many think of yoga as a purely physical practice, the postures were actually developed to help strengthen and stretch the body and prepare it to be able to sit for long periods of time in order to meditate. If the idea of staying still is difficult for you, I suggest getting your willies out first with a good yoga class or other type of exercise, then using a five-minute still meditation as your cool-down.

Resetting your expectations around meditation can help you do it more often, eliminating the pressure or stress many people feel around the practice. If you're new to meditation, I recommend starting small by practicing five to ten minutes every day, beginning with a simple breathing exercise: Inhale slowly for a count of four, then exhale slowly for a count of six.

This will ground you in the present and help bring your body and brain into a state of relaxation. You don't need to close your eyes, sit down, or be in a special mediation room: You can practice this exercise while standing in your office, on a packed subway, or while driving to work. And you don't have to have an epiphany: Just breathe.

If you like the idea of a breathing practice as a way into meditation, you can experiment with doing a four-part breath, or "box breath": Inhale for a count of four, hold for a count of four, exhale for a count of four, then hold for a count of four. At Parsley Health, we do box breaths for two minutes at the start of every executive meeting to ground the session, reduce stress, and bring everyone out of their busy heads and into the room.

The thing about meditation, too, is that you don't ever have to go it alone: You can use breathing apps like Breathe+ Simple Breath Trainer to help guide you, in addition to any of the dozens of meditation-specific apps on the market. I've listed my top five favorite apps below, but definitely experiment to find what's right for you. You can also take meditation classes, in person or virtually—I've listed five of my favorite online teachers if you're interested in trying virtual sessions. Just remember that no teacher or app is better than any other; the best one for you is the one you'll turn to again and again.

DR. BERZIN'S RESOURCE GUIDE TO MEDITATION

My top five favorite meditation apps
Calm
Insight Timer
Headspace
Breathe+ Simple Breath Trainer
10% Happier

My top five favorite meditation books
The Power of Now by Ekhart Tolle
Radical Acceptance by Tara Brach

Letting Go by David R. Hawkins
10% Happier by Dan Harris
Don't Just Sit There! by Biet Simkin

My top five favorite meditation teachers you can find online

David Gandelman (mediationschool.us)
Emily Fletcher (zivameditation.com)
Tara Brach (tarabrach.com)
Jack Kornfield (jackkornfield.com)
Sarah Blondin (sarahblondin.com)

There are dozens of different types of meditation, including transcendental meditation, kundalini, and Vipassana. All of these can work—just like exercise, it's a matter of finding which one makes you feel the best and that you'll want to keep doing. The only meditation to avoid is any that claims it's the only show in town or that charges an exorbitant amount.

After a few weeks of meditating for five to ten minutes daily, you can increase the duration of your sessions if you feel comfortable. Personally, while I know I benefit more the longer I meditate, I don't sit for hours every day. Instead, I try to meditate twenty minutes daily, with one thirty-to-sixty-minute session weekly.

If you're stuck at the five-to-ten-minute mark and don't feel like increasing the duration after a few weeks, I'd recommend you try to expand your practice in other ways. Try guided meditation, whether through an app or a live class, or any number of the topical meditations now available on YouTube and Spotify, including those to help you sleep, recover from a bad breakup, lose weight, prepare for an exam or presentation, better deal with the death of a loved one, or even increase your chances of getting pregnant. Meditating with other people can also heighten the experience in a positive way—many find it's nice to feel part of a community while trying something new like meditation.

HOW TO TAKE MEDITATION TO THE NEXT LEVEL

If you're experienced with meditation and want to deepen your practice, there are many ways to do so. You can try transcendental meditation, which requires a multiday training session and relies on unique silent mantras that you focus on while seated with your eyes closed for twenty minutes, twice per day. If you have the time and opportunity, you can also take a five-to-ten-day silent meditation retreat, which can reset your mind for months or even years to come. (Those with a serious mental health condition should consult with a licensed therapist before signing up for a silent retreat, since the experience will remove you from your support network.) If you don't want to make an extensive investment or time commitment, you can try holotropic breathwork, which involves taking quick, shallow breaths, mimicking hyperventilation, to help trigger a heightened state of calm and mindfulness. You shouldn't do holotropic breathing on your own—look for a qualified instructor who teaches online or in person at a yoga center, spa, or wellness clinic near you.

New Frontier #2: Psychedelic Medicines

I want to start with Psychedelics 101, because I bet most people don't know what they think they know about these psychoactive substances. Psychedelics are a class of hallucinogenic chemicals that shift serotonin activity in the brain, causing altered states of consciousness. There are many different psychedelics and psychedelic-related compounds, but the best-known examples are magic mushrooms (active compound psilocybin), ayahuasca, peyote, ketamine, MDMA (known as ecstasy or molly), and LSD. Psychedelics like mushrooms and peyote are made solely from plants and have been used for centuries by ancient cultures. Synthetic psychedelics like LSD, MDMA, and ketamine were first manufactured in labs in the 1900s, solely for medicinal reasons. It wasn't until the 1960s and '70s that the drugs became widely used for recreational purposes, and subsequently were regulated out of medicinal use.

Before the counterculture era of the mid-twentieth century, psychedelics were extensively studied by public health institutions, including the US government, for their medicinal use in the treatment of mood disorders like depression, anxiety, addiction, and what is now called post-traumatic stress disorder (PTSD). As the cultural backlash around drugs deepened in the 1970s, culminating with the now infamous War on Drugs, psychedelics became heavily regulated, and research on their medicinal use all but stopped. It wasn't until the early 2000s that scientists began studying psychedelics again for medicinal purposes, with Johns Hopkins University becoming the first institution in the US to win approval for clinical trials using the drugs. Since then, organizations like the Multidisciplinary Association for Psychedelic Studies (MAPS), Imperial College London, and New York University have created programs to research how psychedelics can be used to treat mental health conditions.

The results of these clinical trials to date have been impressive. A recent study from Johns Hopkins, for example, found that half of twenty-four participants with major depressive disorder were in remission after taking psilocybin (magic mushrooms) just twice over the course of one month—once in the first week of the trial and the second time in the last week of the trial. Both sessions lasted approximately eleven hours, took place in a clinical setting, and occurred alongside supportive psychotherapy.

While social stigma around psychedelics still exists and many have been slow to embrace the drugs as the next frontier for mental health, the research on their efficacy to help treat mood disorders is promising, to say the least. Here's what we know to date about the three psychedelics with the most clinical research for mood disorders: magic mushrooms, MDMA, and ketamine.

Magic mushrooms (aka psilocybin): Magic mushrooms, with the active compound psilocybin, have been shown to help cure serious cases of depression, oftentimes in instances where drugs and talk therapy had failed, with one study finding the drug reversed major depressive disorder in half of all participants in just one month's time. Other compelling research has shown psilocybin can effectively treat anxiety, leading to significant reductions in feelings of apprehension, fear, and stress, in addition to helping mediate obsessive-compulsive disorder, alcoholism, nicotine addiction, and even suicidal tendencies. These results don't appear to be ephemeral, either: One study found that cancer patients with anxiety and depression had an 80 percent reduction in mental health symptoms four years after receiving one dose of psilocybin—a result scientists say is "mind boggling." While the exact mechanisms behind this kind of impact on mood aren't fully known, doctors believe psilocybin increases available serotonin while also rerouting negative-thought circuits in the brain, the latter being something that antidepressants don't do.

Today, the research on psilocybin is so convincing that the FDA started fast-tracking studies on the drug in 2018, when the federal agency designated it a "breakthrough therapy." Despite this development, magic mushrooms still remain illegal almost everywhere in the US, with the exception of Oregon. While states like California look to pass legislation that would decriminalize psilocybin for mental health treatment, alongside other psychedelics like MDMA, those curious about the drug for therapeutic reasons currently need to be part of a clinical trial or find a licensed psychiatrist who has access to the drug.

MDMA: MDMA, short for midomafetamine, is a synthetic hallucinogenic and stimulant that also goes by the names ecstasy, X, and molly. It's important to note that these recreational versions frequently contain other harmful substances in addition to MDMA. Pure MDMA, however, when administered carefully in a controlled setting, has been shown to effectively treat PTSD after several sessions. This is why the FDA designated the drug as a "breakthrough therapy" in 2017, with the possibility of approval for federal use to treat PTSD by 2023. Outside of PTSD, MDMA has been shown to reduce symptoms of depression by increasing production of certain neurotransmitters, like serotonin, after just one session, eclipsing the time prescription antidepressants require to take effect. Studies also show MDMA can treat anxiety, depression, anger, and despair in people with terminal illnesses after just three sessions. Similar to magic mushrooms, MDMA is illegal in almost every state and currently available for therapeutic uses only via participation in a clinical trial or through a psychiatric professional who obtains the drug illegally.

Ketamine: Ketamine is a dissociative drug, meaning it causes users to detach from their surroundings. While now popular as a club drug, ketamine was first developed in the 1960s as an anesthesia and used on battlefields during the Vietnam War. Today, the drug has amassed impressive research that it can treat depression, even seemingly incurable cases, and has been lauded as "the most impressive breakthrough in antidepressant treatment in decades." According to studies, ketamine can reduce symptoms of depression in just hours, or after one intravenous infusion. While scientists don't exactly understand why, they believe ketamine increases the presence of a neurotransmitter known as glutamate between brain cells, boosting cognitive communication and lowering neuroinflammation. The doses used for these effects are often lower than what's found in recreational ketamine, which can trigger a dangerous side effect called a "k-hole," when the user feels on the edge of losing consciousness.

Unlike magic mushrooms and MDMA, there are more direct and legal ways to obtain ketamine. In 2019, the FDA approved a prescription-only ketamine nasal spray to treat depression in patients who don't respond to other prescription medications. Additionally, dozens of ketamine clinics now offer IV infusions, although consistency and screening vary and you'll have to pay out of pocket— usually several hundred dollars per infusion. These drugs are also being administered "off label," which means they're being used for different means than are FDA approved.

All in all, as research continues to mount showing psychedelics can treat mood disorders in novel ways, experts describe the drugs as "the future of mental health," a "gamechanger," and a possible "mental health revolution." Part of the excitement stems from their efficacy, as well as the fact these drugs appear to reverse mental health symptoms in just weeks, compared to the months or years talk therapy and/or prescription antidepressants often take.

Like many doctors, I believe that psychedelics could revolutionize how we treat mental health. But I also know that there are no shortcuts: You can't just pop a psychedelic on your own and expect miracles. You have to do the work and face your demons—this is why integration therapy is critical to success with psychedelics. You have to partner with a psychiatrist or psychologist, take only pure forms of the drugs, ideally in a controlled, clinical, or supportive setting, and follow up afterward with continued therapy to integrate your psychedelic experiences into new thought patterns and behaviors that can actually transform your everyday life. What's more, psychedelics aren't a substitute for any of our core actions: You still need to eat a brain-healing diet, exercise regularly, get consistent sleep, meditate daily, and make sure any and all underlying health issues are addressed if you want to have the State Change that can overhaul your mind and mood.

When you follow this kind of thoughtful process, though, psychedelics can be a powerful tool to reverse mental-health disorders for some people. That's what happened with my patient Michael, who was a father of two in his mid-forties with clinical anxiety, sometimes to the degree that it interfered with his ability to do his job or show up for his kids. He ate right, exercised regularly, slept consistently, had tried a tech detox, and had taken Zoloft with some benefit, but the medication hadn't helped him get to where he wanted to be. He'd also been in therapy for more than fifteen years and felt stuck.

Recently, Michael had the opportunity to take MDMA at the recommendation of his psychologist, and he completed four eight-hour sessions in a supervised setting while also doing integration therapy work in the intervening weeks. Afterward, he told me that the experience of taking MDMA for therapeutic purposes was nothing like the few times he had tried recreational ecstasy in college.

After three months of MDMA-assisted therapy, Michael experienced a near-total resolution of his anxiety. Since then, he's been able to quit Zoloft and now sees his psychologist only periodically. A year later, he's still largely anxiety-free, without any further MDMA treatments or other medications.

New Frontier #3: Energy Work

The human body is a complicated network of organs, arteries, vessels, bones, muscles, joints, tissues, and cells—and energy. Similar to how we have circulatory, musculoskeletal, and organ systems, human beings also have an energy system—a structure known in Eastern medicine as energy meridians, or pathways that conduct electricity throughout the body. Without this electricity, you wouldn't be able to think, feel, and survive, as electric currents constantly pass between cells, producing some one hundred watts when we're at rest—and up to two thousand watts when we're extremely active, like when we sprint. In other words, each of us is basically a walking electrochemical gradient—an energy current in motion— and if this electrochemical gradient were to suddenly short-circuit, our heart would stop beating, our lungs would no longer work, all our other systems would fail, and we'd die.

In Eastern medicine, energy meridians are well mapped, well understood, and well researched. They are studied as critical, structural pathways that, in a way similar to the knowledge of our system of bones and muscles, can be used to treat physical and mental health conditions. In Western medicine, we recognize that energy meridians exist, but we're not trained to leverage them. In my opinion, this is a problem: We know energy or electricity is critical to human function and survival, but in most fields of Western medicine (with the exception of cardiology, which uses electricity to restart and regulate heart rhythm), we ignore how to use energy to help improve health and well-being.

If an energy meridian system doesn't feel as tangible to you as your skin and bones, think of it this way: All of our cells are like little cities, using and producing electricity to convert the oxygen we breathe and food we eat into energy for our bodies. If the electricity is slow or blocked to these cellular cities, they can't function properly, just like brick-and-mortar cities would fall into decline if someone pulled the power plug. Signs that your energy meridians or electrical grid may be slowed, impaired, or blocked include brain fog, chronic fatigue, ringing in the ears, lethargy, and an immune system that's slow to heal from injury or infection.

As a functional doctor, I've been trained in the value of energy work. The body's autonomic nervous system, responsible for our fight-or-flight response, gets overstimulated and ceases to respond properly to normal stimuli over time, causing our energy meridian system to overload. This, in turn, can lead to mental and emotional instability, along with digestive problems, blood sugar issues, and heart rate irregularities. Energy therapies, which include biofeedback, reiki, craniosacral therapy, massage, and acupuncture, leverage our energy meridians and electrical networks to initiate a healing response.

Energy work can help treat a number of conditions and may be particularly beneficial to those with chronic fatigue, anxiety, insomnia, depression, or other long-lasting mental health disorders. Energy work can also be transformative for those who've been through a physical or emotional trauma, like a car accident, cancer diagnosis, job loss, or the death of a loved one by helping them process the emotional burden instead of holding on to it.

Whether you have a chronic mood condition, have suffered a trauma, or are trying to attain optimal well-being, energy work can help reboot your body's electrical gradient. Unlike surgery or prescription medications, energy work isn't one and done, though: You'll likely need to complete multiple sessions of any one therapy, and you'll definitely need to combine the work with core actions like a brain-healing diet, sleep, and exercise.

There are many different types of energy work, each of which has its own merits. For mood disorders, though, I find the following five to be the most effective:

Biofeedback therapy: Biofeedback therapy uses electrical devices and sensors to help people better understand and control certain physical functions, including the body's brain waves, respiration rate, blood pressure, heart rate, temperature, and muscle contractions. When you receive biofeedback, clinicians attach sensors to your skull, chest, or muscles and use electroencephalography (EEG), electrocardiography (ECG), or a similar electrical-monitoring technology to show you what's happening inside you at different times. Biofeedback sessions typically last thirty minutes to one hour, as a clinician maps your personal pattern of brain waves, heart rate, or whatever physical function you want to measure. You may be able to see this pattern on a screen in real time or your clinician may share your results afterward while helping you decipher what they mean. Either way, a good clinician will help you use the information over time to train your body or brain to help modify these physical biorhythms in order to improve your health. Using biofeedback, for example, you can learn about your breathing patterns and how you might be able to influence them to help calm your nervous system.

Perhaps the most popular form of biofeedback is a proprietary technique known as HeartMath, which assesses heart rate variability (HRV), or the variations in how quickly your heart beats from second to second. While it may not sound like it, having a high HRV is a good thing: It means your heart rate fluctuates frequently in response to stimuli around you. If you have a high HRV, for example, your heart will beat faster if you're approached by a stranger with a knife in a dark alley, but will also slow rapidly after you realize that stranger is actually a friend bearing a bottle of wine. If you have a high HRV, your heart will also speed up or slow down in response to things happening inside your body that you can't consciously feel or perceive. Those with a low HRV, on the other hand, don't have a heart that will beat significantly faster or slower in response to things happening both outside and inside their bodies. While you wouldn't be able to physically feel if you have a low HRV, if you're constantly stressed, anxious, or in a state of fight-or-flight, there's a good chance your HRV is low. Research shows people with a low HRV are at a greater risk for worsening depression and anxiety. HeartMath can teach you how to increase your HRV through various exercises, ultimately retraining your autonomic nervous system and improving your mood.

I typically recommend biofeedback to those with chronic stress or anxiety, a history of eating disorders, a history of trauma, or who feel stuck in a state of fight-or-flight. To find out which type of biofeedback might benefit you the most, consult with a clinician or biofeedback therapy center.

Reiki: Reiki is a Japanese form of medicine in which practitioners use their hands to channel external electrical currents into a patient's body to help shift their internal energy. The technique, also known as energy healing, involves a light touch or no touch at all and relies on the practitioner channeling electrical currents in the world around us, making it much different from massage, which uses varying degrees of touch without attempting to harness external energy currents.

For people in a constant state of fight-or-flight, reiki can be a powerful tool to calm the body and help it relax and heal. Studies show reiki can improve HRV, soothe the autonomic nervous system, and lower feelings of depression, anxiety, stress, and chronic pain. For optimal results, be sure to find a certified practitioner with experience treating mood disorders.

Craniosacral therapy and massage: Craniosacral therapy (CST) and massage are two types of bodywork that rely on human touch to reset energy imbalances in the body. In CST, practitioners apply gentle pressure to the joints of the skull column using their hands, helping to increase flow of cerebrospinal fluid and trigger a state of relaxation. Similarly, massage uses varying degrees of pressure to help relieve tension and energy trapped in muscle, tissue, and fascia.

There are many different types of massage work, including Swedish massage, which uses long, sweeping strokes to help relieve muscle tension, along with deep-tissue massage, which relies on more intense pressure to break up scar tissue in muscle and relax tight connective tissue. Another popular massage technique is Thai massage, which is often performed while the patient is clothed, as a therapist helps stretch out his or her body. In my opinion, the best type of massage for you is the one that feels best, physically, mentally, and emotionally, and that you believe you reap the most lasting benefits from.

No matter which type of massage you prefer or whether you opt for body massage or CST, both therapies harness the healing power of human touch to help soothe the autonomic nervous system, relax muscles, improve circulation, and relieve energy blockages.

In particular, studies show CST can reduce depression and anxiety while improving overall well-being. Massage has also been found to help treat depression, anxiety, fatigue, sleep disorders, and other mood conditions while reducing stress, anger, and irritability. According to research, both therapies help improve headaches, migraines, and chronic pain, while massage may also reduce the risk of chronic disease. Personally, I aim to get a massage every two weeks. Afterward, I always feel a sense of lightness and prolonged relaxation, and both therapies have become part of my energetic maintenance mode, necessary to help reset my energy in a hectic life.

In many areas of the world, massage isn't considered a luxury like it is here in the US but is viewed as imperative to basic health. There are ways, however, to make massage and CST more cost-effective in the States: Look for either at physical therapy clinics or university training programs, which often offer less expensive forms of the treatment. Additionally, some health insurance policies will cover massage or CST if you have a certain medical condition.

I recommend CST and/or massage to those with chronic stress, fatigue, anxiety, a history of trauma, or who can't relax no matter what they do. You don't necessarily need both, although it is possible to find therapists trained in the two techniques. I suggest you experiment to see which one is most effective for you. Just be sure to do either consistently for at least a month before deciding whether the therapy is right for you.

Acupuncture: The best-known and most well-established form of energy work, acupuncture has been used for more than two thousand years in China and other parts of Asia. The practice, which inserts hyper-thin needles into specific points of the body to stimulate improved energy flow and release blockages, has reams of research corroborating its effectiveness in treating a number of conditions—which is why the practice is now covered by many health insurance policies for mood disorders like insomnia, anxiety, and depression, in addition to physical problems like chronic pain, infertility, and irritable bowel syndrome. Studies show acupuncture can help treat depression and anxiety as effectively as psychiatric drugs in some instances, as well as chronic fatigue, sleep disorders, ADHD, and cognitive impairment. Research has also found acupuncture may increase the efficacy of some prescription antidepressants. In my practice, I've seen acupuncture work beautifully for many patients. One of my moms, for example, developed adrenal fatigue after her eight-year-old daughter, Clara, stopped sleeping through the night. Clara was well past the age when young children typically suffer sleeping difficulties, but she had developed childhood anxiety, which kept her up at night—and for which her pediatrician recommended prescription drugs to treat both the girl's insomnia and her anxiety. My mom patient wasn't comfortable putting her young daughter on these drugs, which can cause a host of side effects even in adults, so she sent her daughter to a licensed acupuncturist after another mom recommended the technique. After just one session, Clara had noticeably less anxiety, and after five sessions, the girl was sleeping soundly through the night, as was her mom, my patient.

I prescribe acupuncture to those with musculoskeletal problems, digestive issues, and hormonal imbalances, in addition to chronic stress or anxiety. Just like all the energy work detailed here, it's necessary to work with a licensed therapist on a regular basis for at least several weeks before deciding if acupuncture is beneficial for you.

*

Many of the new frontiers, as it turns out, are actually quite old, combining ancient understandings of the human body and plant medicine with modern research. Because these tools are outside the industrial pharmaceutical realm, conventional medicine largely discounts them—much to everyone's detriment. I believe we should take advantage of all the tools in our toolkit to feel better. Prescription medications are a critical part of the solution, but they aren't the only part—and too often, they're not enough. If you're seeking greater energy flow and peace than modern life or modern medicine affords, looking outside the box to these frontier therapeutics may be the path to a State Change.

CHAPTER TEN

Putting Words to Work:
A Thirty-Day Plan to Reset Your Mind and Mood

The path to success is to take massive, determined actions.

I didn't say that—the famous motivational speaker and author Tony Robbins did. And it couldn't be more relevant to your life right now: Learning how to change your health and actually implementing those changes are distinctly different things. You can read this entire book and intellectually grasp all the information, but if you don't do anything, you won't get better. You have to take determined actions if you want to turn learning into success and change your mind and mood.

At Parsley Health, we're all about outcomes. We don't just want to test and prescribe: What we really care about is making sure our patients get better and achieve the sustained physical and mental health results they want. That's what it means to create a State Change: You have to change something about your current situation in order to shift something about your future situation. And change requires action.

In this chapter, I'm going to show you how to take that action by detailing two thirty-day courses to create true State Changes in your life: a kickstarter plan to begin your journey from the strongest position and an advanced plan for when you're ready to go to the next level. Both plans provide a clear, accessible path to the thoughtful, determined actions that will lead you to success. If you follow either plan closely, I guarantee you will shift your mind and mood.

For the majority of readers, the kickstarter plan is the best place to start. The kickstarter plan combines the essential medical testing and key core actions outlined in this book in a way that is accessible and extremely doable. No matter where you are in your journey to good health, the kickstarter plan can help you reach a new baseline of greater steady-state health and happiness. And for many, thirty days of the kickstarter plan will initiate a powerful State Change.

The advanced plan is more rigorous than the kickstarter plan; it includes more investigative medical testing and a deeper commitment to the key core actions outlined in this book. This plan is designed for those who have followed the core actions in the book on a near-daily, consistent basis; those who have a chronic illness or receive a high score on the Parsley Symptom Index (PSI); or those who've already completed the kickstarter plan and want to take their well-being to the next level.

Both the kickstarter and advanced plans are designed to be supportive. They aren't meant to cure major depressive disorders, schizophrenia, or other serious mental health conditions, or take the place of medication. That said, after working with thousands of patients who have adopted these plans, I know they can help you jump to the next level of mental well-being and experience the State Change we're all capable of.

What to Do Before Starting a Plan

Before you begin either plan, I recommend you take or retake the PSI on pages 32–39 if it's been more than two weeks since you completed it. The PSI will help you establish a baseline for your current health and identify which symptoms are your prevailing hot spots. The PSI can also show you if you have physical symptoms, like digestive difficulties or musculoskeletal pain, that are traveling alongside your mental symptoms. Additionally, the PSI will let you track your progress when you redo the score after one month, which allows you to see exactly how much and in which ways your physical and mental health improved with the adoption of the plan. I don't recommend relying on memory to recall how you felt before you started a plan: most people, including myself, can't remember what they had for lunch last Tuesday, let alone what they felt like last week or four weeks ago.

Taking the PSI can also help you decide which plan to pick: If your PSI score is higher than 75, you likely have several symptoms across different body systems, which often means you have a chronic disease or multiple underlying illnesses. In this case, you can still start with the kickstarter plan if you haven't tried changing your core actions in the past—it's safe to follow, and you will see benefits. But no matter which plan you pick, you should also see a doctor if your PSI score is higher than 75, as we can't do this journey alone—we all need support.

In addition to the PSI, I highly recommend you take or retake the self-assessment on pages 62–63 if you haven't completed it in the past two weeks. The self-assessment will help you identify which core actions you're already taking, which ones you might need to do more regularly, and which ones you'll need to adopt as new behaviors. The self-assessment can also help you determine which plan is right for you: If you're doing at least 80 percent of the core actions specified in the assessment on a near-daily basis, I'd recommend adopting the advanced plan.

Pro tip: The self-assessment only works when you're *honest* with yourself. Lots of patients tell me they've tried going gluten-free, they don't eat sugar, they exercise regularly, or they otherwise lead a healthy lifestyle. But when we start to dig into the details, we discover that they tried going gluten-free one week several years ago, they consume more sugar than they think they do, they aren't moving their bodies long or consistently enough, or they simply aren't as healthy as they thought they were. The core actions outlined in this book, including eating a plant-based paleo diet, moving your body in meaningful ways on a regular basis, and getting enough quality sleep are "core" for a reason: They should be central in your life. If these actions are a "sometimes" rather than an "always," other actions you take to improve your eneergy and flow may not yield the full results that they could. It's like taking an antidepressant every once and in a while—it's probably not going to work. You need to take the medication daily to see improvements in your mind and mood. In this case, the medication is the foods, movements, supplements, and other core actions we've outlined throughout the book.

As a mother and CEO, I don't always eat super-clean, exercise can slip out of my schedule, and I can get overwhelmed by screens, especially since the start of the COVID-19 pandemic. But when I follow the kickstarter plan, I feel significantly better and experience the consistent kind of State Change, with more calm, positive outlook, focus, energy, and even flow, that is palpable and real to me. In other words, there's no shade in getting a kickstart, even if you're the most wellness-savvy person.

Second pro tip: No matter which plan you pick, you don't have to stop at thirty days. Both plans are designed to form the foundation of a lifestyle, and everything I recommend can be done regularly and consistently, with the exception of medical testing and certain intensive experiences in the advanced plan like psychedelics and silent meditation retreats.

One last note: Both plans advocate getting certain medical tests, which require access to a regular primary care doctor, or in the case of the advanced plan, a functional or integrative doctor who is trained to order and interpret more in-depth testing. While I suggest completing diagnostic testing before or shortly after starting either plan, if you don't have access to a doctor or a clear path for medical testing, don't let it block you from beginning the kickstarter plan and adopting the core actions that can help you experience a State Change in a matter of weeks.

HOW TO DO ANYTHING FOR THIRTY DAYS

- **Just do it, now.** I can tell you right now that there's no good time or magic day of the month when it will be convenient for you to start to make these changes. If you keep waiting for the right time, you'll never do it. We're all busy, we all have stuff going on. Start now and don't look back.

- **Own your power in the problem.** You didn't create your mind and mood issues, and they aren't your fault, but they are here. Now it's up to you and you only to create the mood, mind, and life you want. Anything's possible when you stop making excuses and start taking action.

- **Start slowly.** If it feels too challenging to adopt all the core actions specified by the plan at once, introduce them in day-by-day increments over the first week: Eliminate the recommended foods the first day you start the plan, start to take supplements the second day, add exercise the third day, adopt the suggested tech modifications the fourth day, and so on.

· **Head online for inspiration.** If you want recipes for the elimination diet or need ideas to do cardio, stress-relieving, or strength-building workouts at home, head to the Parsley Health blog at parsleyhealth.com/library and following @parsleyhealth on Instagram and Facebook. You'll find dozens of recipes, videos, and articles on how to optimize your health that can help inspire you and keep you committed.

The Kickstarter Plan

Get tested. No matter who you are or what symptoms you have, everyone should get the following thirteen simple blood tests on an annual basis—no exceptions. These tests are part of routine blood work (or should be), require a single blood draw, can be ordered by any doctor, and are covered by health insurance. If you haven't received all thirteen tests in the past year, make an appointment to see your doctor. By now, you know well that mood isn't just in your mind but also in your body, which is why it's so important to make sure a physical condition isn't causing or worsening mood instability. While you can absolutely begin the kickstarter plan without medical testing, you may not see the success you want if you happen to have a blood sugar imbalance, high inflammation, a nutrient deficiency, or a thyroid issue you don't know about. If testing reveals an underlying condition, work with your doctor to address it. Refer back to Chapter Four for more information on the benefits of these tests:

- Three blood sugar tests: HgBA1C, fasting glucose, and fasting insulin
- Three inflammation tests: hsCRP, ESR, and ANA
- Three thyroid tests: TSH, free T4, and free T3
- Four tests for nutrient deficiencies: Vitamin D_3, vitamin B_{12}, RBC-folate, and ferritin

Eliminate these four inflammatory food groups for thirty days. You'll never know how good you can possibly feel if you continue to feed your body

THE KICKSTARTER PLAN SNAPSHOT

Get tested.

⁕ Ask your doctor to test your blood levels of TSH, free T4, free T3, fasting glucose, fasting insulin, HgBA1C, vitamins D_3 and B_{12}, RBC-folate, ferritin, hs-CRP, ANA, and ESR.

Adopt the thirty-day elimination diet.

⁕ Drop all gluten, dairy, added sugars, and processed foods for one month.

Begin the Supplement Starter Kit.

⁕ Take methylated B_{12} and methyl-folate (5MTHF), 1,000 mcg of each daily.

⁕ Take omega-3 fatty acids (EPA/DHA), 1,300 mg daily.

⁕ Take vitamin D_3 with K2, 5,000 IU daily.

⁕ Take high-quality probiotics daily.

Move meaningfully.

⁕ Do twenty minutes of aerobic exercise two days per week.

⁕ Do forty-five minutes of controlled movement (e.g., yoga, tai chi, qigong) two days per week.

* Do twenty minutes of strength building two days per week.

* Do one day of rest and chill per week.

🕐 **Rethink your bedtime.**

* Go to bed by ten p.m. every night to limit evening cortisol spikes.

📶 **Control your tech.**

* Place a one-hour daily time limit on all social media, and shut down all screens by nine p.m.

🧘 **Meditate.**

* Meditate or practice controlled breathing exercises for at least five minutes per day.

THE ADVANCED PLAN SNAPSHOT

🔬 **Make an appointment with a functional doctor.**

  * Ask for all tests outlined in the Kickstarter Plan, in addition to anti-thyroid peroxidase antibody, antithyroglobulin antibody, a five-point cortisol test, estrogen, progesterone, testosterone, DHEA, MTHFR variant, COMT variant, magnesium, selenium, iodine, zinc, and omega-3 index. If applicable, consider an antidepressant pharmacological assessment; tests for Lyme disease, Epstein-Barr virus, and/or toxic mold; and a hydrogen/methane breath and/or three-day stool test.

🥑 **Adopt a *strict* thirty-day elimination diet.**

  * Drop all gluten, dairy, added sugars, processed foods, alcohol, and grains for one month.

💊 **Personalize your supplements.**

  * Take the Supplement Starter Kit as outlined in the Kickstarter Plan, *and*

Take one of the following additional supplements, choosing based on the issue you want to address first:

  * Take ashwagandha and Schisandra for anxiety, 200–400 mg each daily, *or*

* Take magnesium glycinate or magnesium threonate for sleep, 200–400 mg or 1 gm daily, respectively, before bed, *or*

* Take a blend of GABA and L-theanine for insomnia, 600–800 mg and 100–200 mg of each, respectively, daily before bed, *or*

* Take St. John's wort, 5-HTP, *or* SAMe for depression, 300 mg, 100 mg, or 100 mg, respectively, daily, *or*

* Take *Rhodiola rosea* for low energy, 100–200 mg twice daily.

👟 **Move even more meaningfully.**

* Incorporate aerobic, controlled, and strength building movement into your workouts every week, focusing on the one you may be most reluctant to do.

* Increase the intensity or duration of the type of movement you enjoy doing the most.

🕐 **Dissect your sleep.**

* Go to bed by ten p.m. every night to limit evening cortisol spikes.

*   Use a sleep tracker to monitor your sleep metrics.

*   Get tested for sleep apnea if applicable.

📶 **Do a thirty-day digital detox.**

*   Avoid all social media and news platforms for one month.

🧘 **Deepen your meditation.**

*   Meditate for at least twenty minutes daily.

*   Consider regular meditation classes or a meditation retreat.

🔍 **Explore the next frontier.**

*   Talk with a licensed clinician about whether psychedelic drug therapy might be right for you.

*   Experiment with energy work, including biofeedback, reiki, acupuncture, massage, and craniosacral therapy.

toxic crap. Sorry to be blunt, but it's true. While not everyone has a problem with dairy and gluten, processed foods and added sugars will slow you down and prevent you from feeling your best, no matter who you are. What's more, if you have a sensitivity or intolerance to dairy or gluten, it is likely causing or worsening your mood issues.

For these reasons, everyone should give up the following four food groups for thirty days: processed foods, and anything with added sugar, gluten, and dairy. For more information on why and how to do a thirty-day elimination diet, see Chapter Six.

For many, doing an elimination diet will be the biggest hurdle of the plan. To help you stay committed, remind yourself that you only need four weeks to ascertain just how good you can feel for the rest of your life. What's more, you won't starve, and you don't have to "diet." Newsflash: This is *not* about weight loss, though some people do lose weight on the plan as their bodies release inflammation. Instead, you will be eating a ton of delicious foods that fuel your body for peak physical, mental, and emotional performance. You'll get to enjoy things like fresh vegetables and fruits, beans and legumes, seafood, nuts, gluten-free grains, and grass-fed beef and chicken. See pages 155–57 for suggested foods to eat during the thirty-day elimination diet.

On the kickstarter plan, you should also limit your alcohol consumption to no more than three times per week. This plan won't work if you're pouring too much of a known toxin and depressant into your body most days of the week.

After thirty days, introduce gluten or dairy (but not both at once) back into your diet to see if your symptoms return—see Chapter Six for more information on how to reintroduce foods. As for processed foods and added sugars, try to limit your consumption as much as possible after the thirty-day plan ends. This should be easier to do now that you've reset your palate, and the longer you avoid them, the less you'll crave them.

Start the Supplement Starter Kit. In Chapter Eight, you learned about the Supplement Starter Kit, which includes the four dietary supplements I think everyone should take on a daily basis, regardless of their health or mood issues. On the kickstarter plan, I want you to begin the Starter Kit, which has been proven to boost energy and focus, support optimal cognitive function, and shift your gut microbiome to attain a healthier balance. As always, if you start something and you don't feel well, stop it and talk to your doctor, and read ingredients lists to ensure there aren't any ingredients to which you have known allergies.

- Methylated B_{12} and methylated folate (5MTHF), 800–1,000 mcg of each daily
- Marine omega-3 fatty acids, 1,300 mg daily (800 mg EPA, 500 mg DHA)
- Vitamin D_3 with K_2, 5,000 IU daily
- Probiotics, 1–2 capsules daily, as directed

Begin moving meaningfully. Moving your body more in any way possible on a regular basis can help you have a State Change, especially if you're sedentary or exercise only sporadically. But if you want to be efficient about moving your body in a targeted way to boost your mood—or you've been working out for years and still aren't where you want to be—I recommend adopting the following exercise prescription, detailed in Chapter Five. My workout prescription combines three different types of physical activity—aerobic exercise, controlled movement, and strength building—each of which serves a distinct purpose to help prevent and treat anxiety, burnout, and fatigue:

- 2 days x 20 minutes of aerobic exercise per week
- 2 days x 45 minutes of controlled movement per week (e.g., yoga, tai chi, qigong)
- 2 days x 20 minutes of strength building per week
- 1 day rest and chill per week

If starting with six days of movement feels like a lot, I get it. Ease the transition by making it your goal to walk twenty to thirty minutes three days per week—this will get you outside, moving, and out of your stagnant routine. Three other days of the week, make a point to try to check out the three types of activities described here, whether you choose to do gentle yoga, strength-build with resistance bands, or take an online cardio class. If it still feels overwhelming, you don't have to complete the exercises for the time recommended. You also don't need a gym or special membership: Look online for videos of cardio classes, yoga, tai chi, and qigong and build strength by investing in inexpensive resistance bands or home weights.

Go to bed no later than 10 p.m., no matter when you get up. Whether you want to have a State Change or just ensure your body has the daily opportunity to rest, repair, and heal, you'll need to get consistent, high-quality sleep—period. There's no way to cheat this by drinking more caffeine, popping supplements, or making up for missed sleep on the weekends.

The best way to get consistent, high-quality sleep is to go to bed at the same time every night, which will help retrain your body to release melatonin and induce sleepiness when needed. But I want you to take it one step further for thirty days and go to bed at or before 10 p.m., regardless of when you have to get up the next morning. The time of 10 p.m. isn't arbitrary: It lets your body avoid the nighttime spike in cortisol that occurs around midnight, giving you a second wind and interfering with your body's ability to sleep or reach deep sleep. What's more, most people staying up past 10 p.m. are just looking at screens, which will mess with your sleep for all the reasons outlined in Chapter Seven.

Adopt a one-hour daily time limit on social media and shut all screens down at 9 p.m. Most people have no idea just how much time they're spending every day scrolling on Instagram, Facebook, TikTok, news apps, and other digital feeds. Not only can social and news platforms be a huge time suck, they can also damage your mental health by triggering feelings of insecurity, envy, isolation, anxiety, and even fear. Too much media also prevents you from connecting with people in real life, exercising, pursuing hobbies, and enjoying other IRL experiences that have been shown to boost self-esteem, community, and feelings of joy.

To get your social media habit under control, set a total time limit on all your digital-feed apps of no more than one hour a day for the next thirty days—see Chapter Seven for more information on how and why to do this. Use the hour you gain back every day to pursue analog activities like cooking, reading, exercising, socializing, or meditating.

If you don't use social media or look at news feeds that often, this step may not help you shift your mental health. Instead, try cutting down on your total screen time to see if it makes a difference in how you feel. You can also consider adopting a thirty-day tech detox in the advanced plan, in which you eliminate all social media and online news for this month.

Finally, shut down your devices one hour before bed, powering off your phone, laptop, computer, tablet, and TV at 9 p.m. Avoiding screens one hour before bed will help prevent overstimulation and blue-light exposure that can interfere with sleep quantity and quality.

Meditate or breathe mindfully for at least five minutes per day. Most people live in constant fight-or-flight mode, meaning they're never in a parasympathetic state when their nervous system can just rest, digest, relax, and heal. This can cause or worsen mood issues, in addition to digestive problems, hormone imbalances, and other physical problems. To stop the continual state of fight-or-flight and finally calm your body and brain, do five to ten minutes of meditation or breathing exercises every day—no excuses. Studies show that focusing on your breathing for as little as five to ten minutes can cut stress and stop the repetitive, negative thoughts that lead to emotional instability and burnout.

The Advanced Plan

Start by checking in with a functional medicine doctor for more advanced testing. In Chapter Four, I listed a number of diagnostic tests that, in an ideal world, we'd all get. These include the thirteen essential tests that are part of the kickstarter plan, in addition to: two more thyroid tests (anti-thyroid peroxidase and antithyroglobulin antibodies), a five-point cortisol test, saliva- or urine-based sex-hormone testing (estrogen, testosterone, progesterone, and DHEA), genetic testing (MTHFR variant, COMT variant, and antidepressant pharmacological assessment if applicable), and advanced nutrient testing (magnesium, selenium, iodine, zinc, and omega-3 index). On the advanced plan, I want you to get these tests if you have the means and access to a functional or integrative doctor. This kind of testing can reveal underlying physical issues in the body that are impacting your psychological state.

In addition, if any of the essential immune tests that are part of the kickstarter plan—ANA, ESR, or hsCRP—show elevated inflammation, I also recommend stage-two immunity testing for Lyme disease, Epstein-Barr virus, and toxic mold illness, along with additional autoimmune screening as your doctor deems appropriate. If you have gastrointestinal issues, I also suggest a hydrogen/methane breath test and/or three-day stool test to ascertain possible gut infections or imbalances.

One thing I want to stress: When it comes to these more advanced tests, you will usually need to see a functional or integrative doctor. While conventional physicians can order these tests, typically only a functional or integrative doctor or a specialist has the training and experience to correctly interpret the results and develop an appropriate prescription plan for treatment. You can go to Parsley Health, the largest functionally trained medical group in the country, available online for telehealth-based care nationwide, or search the Institute for Functional Medicine's website, which offers a directory of providers near you. Functional medicine is becoming more and more accessible these days, and most practices accept some form of health insurance, or you can get reimbursed by your health insurance plan with their help.

HELPFUL LINKS TO FIND A FUNCTIONAL DOCTOR

- Parsley Health: https://www.parsleyhealth.com/
- Institute for Functional Medicine: https://www.ifm.org/find-a-practitioner/

Other practices with online services that I recommend:

- Cleveland Clinic Center for Functional Medicine: https://my.clevelandclinic.org/departments/functional-medicine
- Dr. Will Cole: https://drwillcole.com/
- The Morrison Center: https://www.morrisonhealth.com/
- The Ultrawellness Center: https://www.ultrawellnesscenter.com/
- Chris Kresser: https://chriskresser.com/

Functional psychiatrists with online practices whom I recommend:

- Dr. Drew Ramsey: https://drewramseymd.com/
- Dr. Ellen Vora: https://ellenvora.com/

Eliminate these six food groups for thirty days. On the advanced plan, you'll adopt the same thirty-day elimination diet as in the kickstarter plan, but in addition to cutting out processed foods, added sugar, gluten, and dairy, you'll also stop consuming all grains and alcohol entirely for four weeks. While whole grains can be part of a plant-based paleo diet (see page 142 for why), they can also be problematic for some people, triggering blood sugar imbalances and allergen-induced inflammation that can cause or worsen underlying conditions, particularly inflammatory and autoimmune disorders. The best way to determine whether grains pose this kind of problem for you is to cut them out completely for four weeks. If you've tried going gluten-free in the past and didn't see a difference, note that going gluten-free, which means avoiding wheat, rye, spelt, and barley, isn't the same as going grain-free, which also includes rice, quinoa, farro, oats, etc. I've seen patients eliminate all grains from their diet and discover they have a lot more energy, mental clarity, and digestive comfort.

On the advanced plan, I advise that you completely stop drinking alcohol, which is a depressant and can interfere with your blood sugar and sabotage your sleep. Going thirty days without booze can also help you break free of the social dependency and unlock a higher level of emotional stability. If the idea of giving up booze for thirty days is super nerve-wracking, that's a good indicator that you need to break the habit more than ever.

Personalize your supplement routine to your mood. On the advanced plan, take the Supplement Starter Kit, detailed on page 198, which is your foundation for a healthy low-neuroinflammation brain state. From there, you can add specific supplements that can target your specific emotional and energetic goals:

- If you feel on edge or anxious during the day, take a blend of 200–400 mg each of ashwagandha and Schisandra daily, in the morning and evening.

- If you have trouble relaxing at night or can't fall asleep, take 200–400 mg of magnesium glycinate or 1 gm magnesium threonate daily before bed.
- If you have insomnia or wake up in the middle of the night, take a blend of 600–800 mg of GABA and 100–200 mg L-theanine thirty minutes before bed nightly.
- If you have mild depression or low mood, try taking *either* 300 mg St. John's wort, 100 mg 5-HTP, or 200 mg SAMe daily (do not take more than one at a time, and speak to your doctor first if you're on an antidepressant medication; for more information, reread Chapter Eight, on supplements).
- If you have low energy or persistent fatigue, take 100–200 mg of *Rhodiola rosea* with both breakfast and lunch.

If you have multiple goals around energy, outlook, and calm, pick the issue that's the most overwhelming or pressing and take the corresponding supplement for at least three weeks—enough time to assess whether it helps or not. If you see results, keep taking that supplement and only then add another one for a different issue; if you don't see results, try something else altogether. For additional suggestions, revisit Chapter Eight.

If you have cancer, are pregnant or nursing, have liver- or kidney-function issues, are already taking a pharmaceutical drug to address a mood disorder such as an SSRI, or have any other medical condition, consult your doctor before taking any supplements. Remember, too, that no supplement can treat or cure a disease, but they can be supportive in finding your State Change.

Increase the frequency or duration of your mood-boosting movement. For many of you, being really targeted about what kind of movement you do and incorporating cardio, controlled exercise, and strength building into your weekly routine will push your mind and mood to the next level. But if you're already doing these three forms of physical activity for the durations specified on page 106, dial up the duration or frequency of what makes you feel good. If you love hiking, biking, or yoga, for example, bump up the frequency or duration of your sessions of these activities to see if you can reap a bigger benefit. Focus first on frequency: For many, it's not about how long they exercise but how often they do it. I have some patients, for example, for whom their daily cardio class, run, or yoga session is a lifeline—if they don't do it almost every day, they feel out of sorts both mentally and physically. Experiment to see what works best for you. I suggest at least thirty minutes daily of cardio to see max effects, with two sixty-minute sessions weekly.

Dissect your sleep on a deeper level. On the advanced plan, you'll want to go to bed by or before 10 p.m. for the same reasons provided in the kickstarter plan. But if you've been struggling with mental health issues or physical illness for a while or simply want to know how sleep affects your mood, use this month to experiment with sleep trackers like the Oura Ring or Apple Watch. Both can help you understand how your daily activities and nighttime environment may be affecting your sleep patterns.

If you snore or wake up often in the night, I'd also recommend seeing your doctor about a sleep apnea test. Sleep apnea, a potentially dangerous disorder that occurs when your breathing becomes disrupted while you sleep, can cause depression, irritability, and fatigue, in addition to other physical and mental symptoms. While many tend to think sleep apnea affects only older or very overweight people, the disorder is common in those of all ages and builds. If your partner says you snore, or you drink alcohol most nights, or you wake up exhausted even after a full night's sleep, you could have sleep apnea.

Do a full thirty-day tech detox. If you're ready for the advanced plan, you've likely already tried taking steps to shift your mental state. Deleting all social-media and news apps for thirty days may sound extreme, but for many, it's the one thing that unlocks a new level of mental and emotional well-being and allows them to have a State Change. For a reminder of how and why to do a thirty-day tech detox, see Chapter Seven.

Deepen your meditation and relaxation practice. In the kickstarter plan, I recommend five to ten minutes of breathing exercises daily. This is a great starting place, but it's not the ending place. For 99 percent of people, meditating for longer periods of time will be even more beneficial: A consistent, committed meditation practice can be a wonderful way to put your body into a state of healing and discover a higher level of energy, mental clarity, and emotional stability. On the advanced plan, try to do twenty to thirty minutes of breathing exercises or meditation at least three days per week, with at least ten minutes of breathing or meditation the remaining days. From here, you can upgrade to twenty minutes twice a day every day, with a one-hour session weekly, which is my target regimen for optimal mental well-being. Few things fall into the "more is better" category in life, but meditation is one of them, within reason (there's no need to meditate more than sixty minutes daily unless you're taking part in a short-term retreat). And don't be worried about the time it takes to meditate twice daily: Some of the most successful people in the world, including Oprah Winfrey, Jerry Seinfeld, Russell Simmons, hedge-fund manager Ray Dalio, Rupert Murdoch, and many others, claim that meditating twice daily gives them the clarity and focus to be more creative, effective, and efficient.

If you have the time and opportunity, I also suggest a meditation retreat, whether it's for one weekend, one week, or longer. Most people I know who've attended meditation retreats say the experience transformed their lives and allowed them to bring what they learned into their everyday practice with much greater depth. A retreat is a great way to learn how to meditate if you're new to the activity. Or if you've been practicing for years, a retreat will likely help recharge your enthusiasm for or deepen your practice. I've heard from those who've come back from a retreat that they felt the experience finally ended their self-doubt over whether they were meditating the "right" way.

Consider next-frontier therapies like psychedelics and energy work. While psychedelics aren't right for everyone, if you've been suffering with a mood disorder for some time without any mitigation, talk with your psychiatrist or psychologist about whether clinical psychedelic treatment may be right for you. This is *not* something you can DIY, though: You must consult with a trained professional and do the hard work of integration therapy for psychedelics to treat a mood issue. This means finding a licensed professional trained in psychedelic experiences who can help you identify and incorporate into your everyday life any realizations made during your trip. See Chapter Nine for more information.

Finally, no matter who you are or what you're struggling with, almost everyone can benefit from regular energy work, like biofeedback, reiki, acupuncture, massage, and craniosacral therapy, which are all practices that use the body's energy grid to help restore energetic balance and calm the sympathetic nervous system. These therapies are safe, supportive ways to help your body reach a new level of healing and achieve a higher baseline of relaxation.

Capping It Off: Get Your Score and Enjoy the Progress You've Made

No matter which plan you follow, the most important thing to do after you finish is retake the PSI on pages 32–39 to assess how you feel and what's changed over the last thirty days. The PSI can give you an objective and clear measurement of your physical and mental health, which you can compare to your physical and mental health one month prior, allowing you to determine which areas of your body, mind, and emotional state have changed, and which haven't.

If you don't feel any different than you did thirty days ago, you're certainly free to go back to your old baseline habits. But in my experience, my patients who do so ultimately discover that they feel worse after reintroducing sugar or gluten, drinking more alcohol, giving up exercise, increasing their screen time, and/or returning to their old, unhealthy sleep patterns. If you go back to your old ways and start to feel worse, pay attention to what in particular you believe caused the state shift, whether it was consuming certain foods or getting less consistent sleep or something else. The driver or drivers of your worsening outlook can be the starting place for your future efforts, allowing you to reclaim the State Change you just experienced that much faster.

Most people, however, will notice a marked change after thirty days of either plan, even if you didn't do absolutely everything recommended every single day for the entire month—remember, it's about progress, not perfection. But now it's in your power to determine which core actions were the biggest drivers of your State Change, whether it was eliminating specific foods, taking a foundation of supplements, starting to move more, or finally regulating your sleep or tech habits. Many times, more than one core action is responsible for a State Change, and most of us know intrinsically which ones caused us to achieve a higher baseline. My hope is that these core actions—the most impactful ones—become your new normal.

Beyond Thirty Days

The goal of this book isn't to have a State Change for one month but to experience a series of State Changes over and over again. After you determine which core actions can help you reach a new baseline, you can make them as much a part of your everyday life as possible—in other words, you can make your most influential core actions actually core in your life. This doesn't mean that you have to be perfect. You don't have to eat plant-based paleo or exercise 100 percent of the time, every single day, for the rest of your life. For many people, adopting their core actions every day isn't realistic in a world where we're surrounded by too much sugar, tech, and alcohol, and getting too little sleep and movement are almost expected. We all slide off our through line from time to time, and that's okay. But now when you do slide off, you now know exactly what you need to do to get back to your new baseline and have a State Change again.

My ultimate hope for you is that you experience firsthand how much better you can feel by shifting aspects of your daily life that you may never have paid attention to—things that may seem obvious, unimportant, or just "normal" but aren't. I also want you to realize that healing from within is possible. Whether it's 10 percent or 100 percent, we all have room to feel better. Otherwise, if you continue to live in a way that causes burnout and stress every day, you'll continue to live at a much lower baseline of energy, focus, and vitality than you're capable of or deserve. We all have only one life in this body. I want you to understand on a bodily level, not just an intellectual one, just how great you can feel. And once you have your own State Change and experience a new normal, you'll know exactly what to do to get back to feeling really good because you've already done it. And you'll do it again because you want to, not because you have to.

At the end of the day, we all have the power to have many State Changes throughout our lives. A State Change is never one and done—we can find our new gear over and over again, especially when we know we have the tools to get back to feeling good whenever we want. With each turn, you also have the power and possibility to push your levels higher and higher. Clarity, calm, and better physical and mental health aren't only incredible all on their own—they can also help you take steps in life you never thought possible, and open up new worlds, experiences, careers, and relationships you never could have imagined. That's certainly what happened to me.

Start with the body, and heal your mind. Change your physiology to change your psychology. And once you change your psychology, you can change your entire life.

Acknowledgments

My deepest gratitude goes out to all the people who have made this book possible. While my name is on the cover, this book represents the dedication, creativity, intelligence, and guidance of many, all of whom deserve credit for helping to bring what I have to share into the world.

First, thank you to Sarah Toland, my collaborator. I could not have found a better match for my voice, my commitment to evidence-based writing in medicine, or my goal to make this book as accessible and universal as possible. I don't know how you put up with my hectic schedule, but you somehow managed to roll with my crazy life to get this done. I already miss our Sunday afternoon and Tuesday night calls.

Thank you to Brandi Bowles, my agent at United Talent Agency, whose patience knows no bounds. After something like five years of you encouraging me to write a book, waiting to hear what on earth I wanted to write about, introducing me to an infinite number of collaborators, and checking in continually, we did it.

Thank you to my editor, Leah Miller, and the entire team at Simon & Schuster. This book exists because of your vision and your commitment to support the kind of writing that can help people expand their vision of what is possible in the way they live their lives.

Thank you also to my entire team at Parsley Health, in particular the doctors, nurse practitioners, physician assistants, registered nurses, health coaches, care assistants, and member advisors who deliver incredible patient care every day and whose patient stories appear in this book. Thank you to our data and clinical teams who help create and publish the Parsley Symptom Index and other tools that make our medicine truly actionable. Thanks, too, to Courtney Hamilton, our head of communications, and Brooke Travis, our chief marketing officer, for your wisdom and energy in ensuring this book reflects the mission of our organization and appears in the places and for the people who need it the most. Also thank you to Casey Beck, who keeps me organized and on track week after week, quarter after quarter.

Thank you to some of my dearest friends whose journeys with their own books, podcasts, and creative projects have inspired me. Uzo Iweala, Jo Piazza, Gabby Bernstein, David Gandelman, Dhru Purohit, Dr. Mark Hyman, and Dr. Will Cole: Your feedback along the way gave me the confidence to march forward, and your responses to my last-minute texts, calls, questions, and brainstorms were the reassurance I needed.

Thank you to David, my rock. You have always encouraged me to see my own greatest potential, reminded me not to count myself out, and been my greatest collaborator in life for more than a decade. I love you.

Thank you to my patients. Your stories, successes, challenges, tough cases, expected and unexpected diagnoses, resilience, and power to heal are the true reasons this book exists. When you decide to become a doctor, no one tells you that your real training begins after medical school in the conversations and interactions you have with hundreds or even thousands of patients, who keep teaching you every day to be better as long as you practice.

And thank you to my dad, Dr. Neal Friedlander, the OG top doc, whom I think of every time I tell myself, "Robin, just be a good doctor." You are the ultimate role model.

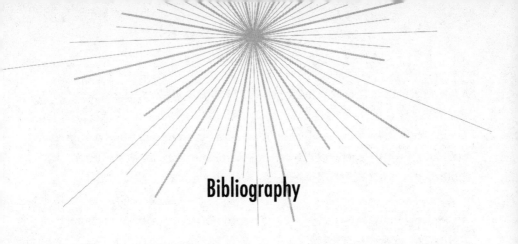

Bibliography

Abuznait, Alaa H., et al. "Olive-Oil-Derived Oleocanthal Enhances β-Amyloid Clearance as a Potential Neuroprotective Mechanism against Alzheimer's Disease: In Vitro and in Vivo Studies." *ACS Chemical Neuroscience* 4, no. 6 (2013): 973–82. https://doi.org/10.1021/cn400024q.

Active Times. "The Surprising Ways Lifting Weights Can Change Your Life." *HuffPost*, April 5, 2015.

"Acupuncture." UCSF Health, October 7, 2020.

"Acupuncture Found Effective for Chronic Fatigue Syndrome." Healthcare Medicine Institute, June 20, 2020.

Adjibade, Moufidath, et al. "Prospective Association between Ultra-Processed Food Consumption and Incident Depressive Symptoms in the French Nutri-Net-Santé Cohort." *BMC Medicine* 17, no. 1 (2019). https://doi.org/10.1186/s12916-019-1312-y.

"A. G. Schneiderman Asks Major Retailers to Halt Sales of Certain Herbal Supplements as DNA Tests Fail to Detect Plant Materials Listed on Majority of Products Tested." Press release. New York State Office of the Attorney General, February 3, 2015.

Aiken, Chris. "Dark Chocolate for Depression." *Psychiatric Times*, September 4, 2019.

Alam, Nuhu, et al. "Comparative Effects of Oyster Mushrooms on Lipid Profile, Liver and Kidney Function in Hypercholesterolemic Rats." *Mycobiology* 37, no. 1 (2009): 37. https://doi.org/10.4489/myco.2009.37.1.037.

Ali, Raian, Emily Arden-Close, and John McAlaney. "Digital Addiction: How Technology Keeps Us Hooked." *Conversation*, January 8, 2021.

Allen, David L., et al. "Acute Daily Psychological Stress Causes Increased Atrophic Gene Expression and Myostatin-Dependent Muscle Atrophy." *American Journal of Physiology—Regulatory, Integrative and Comparative Physiology* 299, no. 3 (2010). https://doi.org/10.1152/ajpregu.00296.2010.

"America's State of Mind: U.S. Trends in Medication Use for Depression, Anxiety, and Insomnia." Express Scripts, April 16, 2020.

American Osteopathic Association. "Low Magnesium Levels Make Vitamin D Ineffective: Up to 50 Percent of US Population Is Magnesium Deficient." Science-Daily, February 26, 2018.

"Americans Sit Almost 10 Hours Each Day (On Average)." On Your Feet America, Accessed May 13, 2021.

Anderson, Pauline. "Sleep Deprivation Leads to Emotional Instability Even in Healthy Subjects." Medscape, July 17, 2020.

Andreone, Benjamin. "Clearing Out the Junk: Healthy Lifestyle Choices Boost Brain Waste Disposal." Science in the News, Harvard University, May 22, 2019.

Arab, Lenore, Rong Guo, and David Elashoff. "Lower Depression Scores among Walnut Consumers in NHANES." *Nutrients* 11, no. 2 (2019): 275. https://doi.org/10.3390/nu11020275.

"Are You Getting Enough Omega-3s?" Institute for Natural Medicine, January 23, 2020.

"Autoimmune Disease Statistics." American Autoimmune Related Diseases Association, 2018.

Azab, Marwa. "Gut Bacteria Can Influence Your Mood, Thoughts, and Brain." *Psychology Today*, August 7, 2019.

Babyak, Michael, et al. "Exercise Treatment for Major Depression: Maintenance of Therapeutic Benefit at 10 Months." *Psychosomatic Medicine* 62, no. 5 (2000): 633–38. https://doi.org/10.1097/00006842-200009000-00006.

Bagherniya, Mohammad, et al. "The Effect of Fasting or Calorie Restriction on Autophagy Induction: A Review of the Literature." *Ageing Research Reviews* 47 (2018): 183–97. https://doi.org/10.1016/j.arr.2018.08.004.

Bahniwal, Manpreet, Jonathan P. Little, and Andis Klegeris. "High Glucose Enhances Neurotoxicity and Inflammatory Cytokine Secretion by Stimulated Human Astrocytes." *Current Alzheimer Research* 14, no. 7 (2017). https://doi.org/10.2174/1567205014666170117104053.

Basso, Julia C., and Wendy A. Suzuki. "The Effects of Acute Exercise on Mood, Cognition, Neurophysiology, and Neurochemical Pathways: A Review." *Brain Plasticity* 2, no. 2 (2017): 127–52. https://doi.org/10.3233/bpl-160040.

Bates, Sophie. "A Decade of Data Reveals That Heavy Multitaskers Have Reduced Memory, Stanford Psychologist Says." *Stanford News*, Stanford University, October 25, 2018.

Bear, Tracey L., et al. "The Role of the Gut Microbiota in Dietary Interventions for Depression and Anxiety." *Advances in Nutrition* 11, no. 4 (2020): 890–907. https://doi.org/10.1093/advances/nmaa016.

Becker, Kate. "Researchers Put Probiotics in Food and Supplements to the Test." Phys.org, November 17, 2017.

Beitsch, Rebecca. "Leaked FDA Study Finds Milk, Meat, Produce Contaminated with 'Forever Chemicals.'" *The Hill*, June 4, 2019.

Berger, M. E., et al. "Omega-6 to Omega-3 Polyunsaturated Fatty Acid Ratio and Subsequent Mood Disorders in Young People with At-Risk Mental States: A 7-Year Longitudinal Study." *Translational Psychiatry* 7, no. 8 (2017). https://doi .org/10.1038/tp.2017.190.

Bier, Deborah. "Reiki Healing and Mental Health: What the Research Shows." Psych Central, May 17, 2016.

Boodman, Sandra G. "For Millennials, a Regular Visit to the Doctor's Office Is Not a Primary Concern." *Washington Post*, October 6, 2018.

Brennan, Dan. "Are There Health Benefits to Using Extra Virgin Olive Oil? Pros and Cons, Nutrition, and More." WebMD, September 30, 2020.

Breselor, Sara. "Sugar High: Why Your Food Is Getting Sweeter." *Salon*, February 15, 2010.

Brewer, J. A., et al. "Meditation Experience Is Associated with Differences in Default Mode Network Activity and Connectivity." *Proceedings of the National Academy of Sciences* 108, no. 50 (2011): 20254–59. https://doi.org/10.1073/pnas.1112029108.

Brooks, David. "How Evil Is Tech?" *New York Times*, November 21, 2017.

Brown, Eileen. "Americans Spend Far More Time on Their Smartphones than They Think." ZDNet, April 28, 2019.

Brown, Mary Jane. "8 Health Benefits of Probiotics." Healthline, 2016.

Brueck, Hilary. "This Is What Your Smartphone Is Doing to Your Brain—and It Isn't Good." *Business Insider*, March 1, 2019.

Budd, Ken. "Keep Your Mental Focus: Older Americans Have Superior Attention Spans." AARP, November 27, 2017.

Burgan, Beth. "How Can Massage Help My Health and Wellbeing?" Taking Charge of Your Health and Wellbeing, University of Minnesota, accessed May 14, 2021.

Cafasso, Jacquelyn. "Endorphins: Functions, Levels, and Natural Boosts." Healthline, July 12, 2017.

Calder, Philip C. "n–3 Polyunsaturated Fatty Acids, Inflammation, and Inflammatory Diseases." *American Journal of Clinical Nutrition* 83, no. 6 (2006). https://doi.org/10.1093/ajcn/83.6.1505s.

"Cancer and Fasting / Calorie Restriction." UCSF Osher Center for Integrative Medicine, University of California San Francisco, 2020.

Canheta, Andrea Batista, et al. "Traditional Brazilian Diet and Extra Virgin Olive Oil Reduce Symptoms of Anxiety and Depression in Individuals with Severe Obesity: Randomized Clinical Trial." *Clinical Nutrition* 40, no. 2 (2021): 404–11. https://doi.org/10.1016/j.clnu.2020.05.046.

Carey, Benedict. "One in 6 American Adults Say They Have Taken Psychiatric Drugs, Report Says." *New York Times*, December 12, 2016. https://www.nytimes.com/2016/12/12/health/one-in-6-american-adults-say-they-have-taken-psychiatric-drugs-report-says.html.

Carpenter, S. "That Gut Feeling." *Monitor on Psychology* 43, no. 8 (September 2012).

Cedars-Sinai Staff. "Is Eating Gluten-Free a Good Idea?" Blog post. Cedars Sinai, May 17, 2018.

"Celiac Disease Facts and Figures." Celiac Disease Center, University of Chicago Medicine, 2021.

Chang, Chia-Yu, Der-Shin Ke, and Jen-Yin Chen. "Essential Fatty Acids and Human Brain." *Acta Neurol Taiwan* 18, no. 4 (December 2009): 231–41.

Chen, Angela. "The FDA Approved a New Ketamine Depression Drug—Here's What's Next." *The Verge*, March 11, 2019.

Chesak, Jennifer. "The No BS Guide to Probiotics for Your Brain, Mood, and Gut." Healthline, March 2020.

Chiu, Chun-Hung, et al. "Erinacine A-Enriched Hericium Erinaceus Mycelium Produces Antidepressant-Like Effects through Modulating BDNF/PI3K/Akt /GSK-3β Signaling in Mice." *International Journal of Molecular Sciences* 19, no. 2 (2018): 341. https://doi.org/10.3390/ijms19020341.

Chodosh, Sara. "Half of the People Who Think They Have Food Allergies Actually Don't." *Popular Science*, January 2019. https://www.popsci.com/allergies-food -intolerances-differences/.

Cojocaru, M., Inimioara Cojocaru, and Isabela Silosi. "Multiple Autoimmune Syndrome." *Maedica: A Journal of Clinical Medicine* 5, no. 2 (2010): 132–34.

Collins, Sonya. "What Is Ketamine? How It Works and Helps Severe Depression." WebMD, 2018.

"Compulsion Loop or Core Loop." Dictionary.com, January 19, 2021.

Cooney, Gary M., et al. "Exercise for Depression." *Cochrane Database of System-atic Reviews* (2013). https://doi.org/10.1002/14651858.cd004366.pub6.

Coppen, Alec, and Christina Bolander-Gouaille. "Treatment of Depression: Time to Consider Folic Acid and Vitamin B_{12}." *Journal of Psychopharmacology* 19, no. 1 (2005): 59–65. https://doi.org/10.1177/0269881105048899.

Corliss, Julie. "Mindfulness Meditation May Ease Anxiety, Mental Stress." Harvard Medical School, January 8, 2014.

Costantini, Lauren C., et al. "Hypometabolism as a Therapeutic Target in Alzheimer's Disease." *BMC Neuroscience* 9, no. S2 (2008). https://doi.org/10.1186/1471 -2202-9-s2-s16.

Creighton University. "Recommendation for Vitamin D Intake Was Miscalculated, Is Far Too Low, Experts Say." ScienceDaily, March 17, 2015.

Crozier, Stephen J., et al. "Cacao Seeds Are a 'Super Fruit': A Comparative Analysis of Various Fruit Powders and Products." *Chemistry Central Journal* 5, no. 1 (2011). https://doi.org/10.1186/1752-153x-5-5.

Dahl, Melissa. "Sleep-Deprived People Can't Tell They're Sleep-Deprived." *The Cut*, July 29, 2014.

Daniel, Jeremy, and Margaret Haberman. "Clinical Potential of Psilocybin as a Treatment for Mental Health Conditions." *Mental Health Clinician* 7, no. 1 (2017): 24–28. https://doi.org/10.9740/mhc.2017.01.024.

Darbinyan, V., et al. "*Rhodiola rosea* in Stress-Induced Fatigue—A Double Blind Crossover Study of a Standardized Extract SHR-5 with a Repeated Low-Dose Regimen on the Mental Performance of Healthy Physicians during Night Duty." *Phytomedicine* 7, no. 5 (2000): 365–71. https://doi.org/10.1016/s0944 -7113(00)80055-0.

Deans, Emily. "Magnesium and the Brain: The Original Chill Pill." *Psychology Today*, June 12, 2011.

"Demographics of Mobile Device Ownership and Adoption in the United States." Pew Research Center, April 26, 2021.

"Depression & Fish Oil/Omega 3 Treatment." WebMD, 2000.

"Depression: How Effective Are Antidepressants?" InformedHealth.org, June 18, 2020.

DiNicolantonio, James J., and James H. O'Keefe. "The Importance of Marine Omega-3s for Brain Development and the Prevention and Treatment of Behavior, Mood, and Other Brain Disorders." *Nutrients* 12, no. 8 (2020): 2333. https://doi .org/10.3390/nu12082333.

Donma, M. M., and O. Donma. "Promising Link between Selenium and Peroxisome Proliferator Activated Receptor Gamma in the Treatment Protocols of Obesity as Well as Depression." *Medical Hypotheses* 89 (2016): 79–83. https://doi .org/10.1016/j.mehy.2016.02.008.

Drake, Victoria. "Micronutrient Inadequacies in the US Population: An Overview." Linus Pauling Institute, January 27, 2021.

Ducharme, Jamie. "Millennials Love Wellness. But They're Not as Healthy as People Think, Report Says." *Time*, April 24, 2019.

———. "Using Your Phone at Dinner Makes You Unhappy, Science Says." *Time*, February 28, 2018.

Duke University Medical Center. "Epstein-Barr: Scientists Decode Secrets of a Very Common Virus That Can Cause Cancer." ScienceDaily, December 15, 2010.

Dunckley, Victoria. "Gray Matters: Too Much Screen Time Damages the Brain." *Psychology Today*, February 27, 2014.

Eby, George A., and Karen L. Eby. "Rapid Recovery from Major Depression Using Magnesium Treatment." *Medical Hypotheses* 67, no. 2 (2006): 362–70. https://doi.org/10.1016/j.mehy.2006.01.047.

Edwards, D., A. Heufelder, and A. Zimmermann. "Therapeutic Effects and Safety of *Rhodiola rosea* Extract WS® 1375 in Subjects with Life-Stress Symptoms—Results of an Open-Label Study." *Phytotherapy Research* 26, no. 8 (2012): 1220–25. https://doi.org/10.1002/ptr.3712.

"Endorphin Release Differs by Exercise Intensity, Study Finds." Medical News Today, accessed May 13, 2021.

Everett, J. M., et al. "Theanine Consumption, Stress and Anxiety in Human Clinical Trials: A Systematic Review." *Journal of Nutrition & Intermediary Metabolism* 4 (2016): 41–42. https://doi.org/10.1016/j.jnim.2015.12.308.

"Exercising for Better Sleep." Johns Hopkins Medicine, 2021.

"Exercising to Relax." Harvard Medical School, July 7, 2020.

Fakorede, Foluso. "Increasing Awareness This National Diabetes Month Can Save Limbs and Lives." AJMC, November 29, 2018.

FCD Prevention Works. "Technology Addiction." Hazelden Betty Ford Foundation, March 16, 2017.

"FDA Approves New Nasal Spray Medication for Treatment-Resistant Depression; Available Only at a Certified Doctor's Office or Clinic." US Food & Drug Administration, March 2019.

Feltman, Rachel. "The FDA Is Fast-Tracking a Second Psilocybin Drug to Treat Depression." *Popular Science*, November 26, 2019.

Fetters, K. Aleisha. "Struggling With Your Mental Health? Get These Nutrient Levels Checked." *U.S. News & World Report*, September 10, 2018.

Fleming, Nic. "Plants Talk to Each Other Using an Internet of Fungus." BBC, November 11, 2014.

Francis, S. T., et al. "The Effect of Flavanol-Rich Cocoa on the FMRI Response to a Cognitive Task in Healthy Young People." *Journal of Cardiovascular Pharmacology* 47, Supplement 2 (2006). https://doi.org/10.1097/00005344-200606001 -00018.

Friday, Francesca. "New Study Reveals Chemical Brain Imbalance in Smartphone Addicts." *Observer*, December 29, 2017.

Gallagher, James. "More Than Half Your Body Is Not Human." BBC, April 10, 2018.

Gao, Qi, et al. "The Association between Vitamin D Deficiency and Sleep Disorders: A Systematic Review and Meta-Analysis." *Nutrients* 10, no. 10 (October 1, 2018): 1395. doi: 10.3390/nu10101395.

Garcia-Navarro, Lulu. "The Risk of Teen Depression and Suicide Is Linked to Smartphone Use, Study Says." NPR, December 17, 2017.

Gariballa, Salah, and Awad Alessa. "Associations between Low Muscle Mass, Blood-Borne Nutritional Status and Mental Health in Older Patients." *BMC Nutrition* 6, no. 1 (2020). https://doi.org/10.1186/s40795-019-0330-7.

"General Information/Press Room." Press release. American Thyroid Association, 2021.

Goldberg, Simon B., et al. "The Experimental Effects of Psilocybin on Symptoms of Anxiety and Depression: A Meta-Analysis." *Psychiatry Research* 284 (2020): 112749. https://doi.org/10.1016/j.psychres.2020.112749.

Gorman, Jack M., and Richard P. Sloan. "Heart Rate Variability in Depressive and Anxiety Disorders." *American Heart Journal* 140, no. 4 (2000). https://doi .org/10.1067/mhj.2000.109981.

Greenwood, Michael T. "Acupuncture, Attention-Deficit Hyperactivity Disorder, and the Energetics of Stimulants." *Medical Acupuncture* 32, no. 1 (2020): 8–15. https://doi.org/10.1089/acu.2019.1395.

Gunnars, Kris. "10 Evidence-Based Health Benefits of Intermittent Fasting." Healthline, August 16, 2016.

Guo, Wanli, et al. "Magnesium Deficiency in Plants: An Urgent Problem." *Crop Journal* 4, no. 2 (April 2016): 83–91.

Guzman, Joseph. "Single Dose of Magic Mushrooms Eases Patients' Anxiety, Depression for Years, New Study Finds." *The Hill*, January 29, 2020.

Hamilton, Jon. "Brains Sweep Themselves Clean of Toxins During Sleep." NPR, October 17, 2013.

Hampton, Debbie. "How Your Thoughts Change Your Brain, Cells and Genes." *HuffPost*, March 24, 2017.

Harrison, Rachel E., and John S. Page. "Multipractitioner Upledger Cranio-Sacral Therapy: Descriptive Outcome Study 2007–2008." *Journal of Alternative and Complementary Medicine* 17, no. 1 (2011): 13–17. https://doi.org/10.1089 /acm.2009.0644.

Heid, Markham. "You Asked: Is Social Media Making Me Miserable?" *Time*, August 2, 2017.

Hellhammer, Juliane, et al. "A Soy-Based Phosphatidylserine/Phosphatidic Acid Complex (PAS) Normalizes the Stress Reactivity of Hypothalamus-Pituitary-

Adrenal-Axis in Chronically Stressed Male Subjects: A Randomized, Placebo-Controlled Study." *Lipids in Health and Disease* 13, no. 1 (2014). https://doi.org/10.1186/1476-511x-13-121.

Holder, Mary K., et al. "Dietary Emulsifiers Consumption Alters Anxiety-like and Social-Related Behaviors in Mice in a Sex-Dependent Manner." *Scientific Reports* 9, no. 1 (2019). https://doi.org/10.1038/s41598-018-36890-3.

"How Meditation Can Help You Focus." Columbia University School of Professional Studies, May 10, 2021.

"How Much Is Too Much?" UCSF Health, December 8, 2018.

"How Is Modern Technology Affecting Human Development?" Walden University, March 25, 2021.

Howard, Jacqueline. "Rates of ADHD Diagnosis among US Adults Are on the Rise, Study Suggests." CNN, November 1, 2019.

Hunt, Katie. "'Magic Mushroom' Ingredient Could Work as Mental Health Treatment." CNN, November 7, 2020.

Hurley, Katie. "Is It Sleep Deprivation or Depression?" Psycom.net, July 21, 2020.

Hyman, Mark. "Maximizing Methylation: The Key to Healthy Aging." DrHyman.com, November 25, 2019.

———. "What NOT to Eat: Part 2." DrHyman.com, October 21, 2019.

———. "Why Vegetable Oils Should Not Be Part of Your Diet." EcoWatch, May 23, 2020.

"Is Sitting All Day Bad for Your Health?" NewYork-Presbyterian, July 17, 2019.

Iyo, Jenny. "Exercise and Insomnia: Can Physical Activity Combat Insomnia?" Sleep Foundation, December 11, 2020.

J. Liu. "Reishi Mushroom." Memorial Sloan Kettering Cancer Center, February 5, 2021.

Jade, Kathleen. "Psychobiotics: Probiotics That May Impact Mood." University Health News Daily, May 13, 2021.

Jangid, Purushottam, et al. "Comparative Study of Efficacy of l-5-Hydroxytryptophan and Fluoxetine in Patients Presenting with First Depressive Episode." *Asian Journal of Psychiatry* 6, no. 1 (2013): 29–34. https://doi.org/10.1016/j.ajp.2012.05.011.

Jedinak, Andrej, et al. "Anti-Inflammatory Activity of Edible Oyster Mushroom Is Mediated through the Inhibition of NF-KB and AP-1 Signaling." *Nutrition Journal* 10, no. 1 (2011). https://doi.org/10.1186/1475-2891-10-52.

Johansson, Anna. "The Chemicals in Your Food Can Affect Your Mood." Thrive Global, October 19, 2017.

Johnson, James B., et al. "Alternate Day Calorie Restriction Improves Clinical Findings and Reduces Markers of Oxidative Stress and Inflammation in Overweight Adults with Moderate Asthma." *Free Radical Biology and Medicine* 42, no. 5 (2007): 665–74. https://doi.org/10.1016/j.freeradbiomed.2006.12.005.

Jones, Taylor. "7 Healthy Foods That Are High in Vitamin D." Healthline, December 18, 2019.

Junghans, Kylee. "Acupuncture as a Therapeutic Treatment for Anxiety." Evidence Based Acupuncture, March 17, 2021.

Kalafatakis, F., et al. "Mobile Phone Use for 5 Minutes Can Cause Significant

Memory Impairment in Humans." *Hellenic Journal of Nuclear Medicine* 20 (2017): 146–54.

Kandola, Aaron A., et al. "Individual and Combined Associations between Cardiorespiratory Fitness and Grip Strength with Common Mental Disorders: A Prospective Cohort Study in the UK Biobank." *BMC Medicine* 18, no. 1 (2020). https://doi.org/10.1186/s12916-020-01782-9.

Kay, Isa. "Is Your Mood Disorder a Symptom of Unstable Blood Sugar?" School of Public Health, University of Michigan, October 21, 2019.

Keegan, Natalie. "Brits Glug Five and Half BATHTUBS of Cooking Oil in Their Lives." *The Sun*, June 13, 2017.

Khalid, Sundus, et al. "Effects of Acute Blueberry Flavonoids on Mood in Children and Young Adults." *Nutrients* 9, no. 2 (2017): 158. https://doi.org/10.3390/nu9020158.

Kim, Hyeong-Geug, et al. "Antifatigue Effects of Panax Ginseng C.A. Meyer: A Randomised, Double-Blind, Placebo-Controlled Trial." *PLoS ONE* 8, no. 4 (2013). https://doi.org/10.1371/journal.pone.0061271.

Knight, Rob. "Social Media Is Getting in the Way of Real-Life Friendships, New Study Claims." *Independent*, February 1, 2019.

Koduah, Priscilla, Paul Friedemann, and Jan-Markus Dörr. "Vitamin D in the Prevention, Prediction and Treatment of Neurodegenerative and Neuroinflammatory Diseases." *EPMA Journal* 8, no. 4 (2017): 313–25.

Kotz, Deborah. "Want to Be Happier? Keep Your Focus." *U.S. News & World Report*, November 2010.

Kravitz Hoeffner, Melissa. "There Are 2,000 Untested Chemicals in Packaged Foods—and It's Legal." *Salon*, November 15, 2019.

Kresser, Chris. "The Fish vs. Fish Oil Smackdown." ChrisKresser.com, May 22, 2010.

Kuyken, Willem, et al. "Efficacy of Mindfulness-Based Cognitive Therapy in Prevention of Depressive Relapse." *JAMA Psychiatry* 73, no. 6 (2016): 565–74. https://doi.org/10.1001/jamapsychiatry.2016.0076.

LaBonta, Lo'eau. "Human Energy Converted to Electricity." Stanford University, December 2014.

"Lactose Intolerance." MedlinePlus, August 18, 2020.

Lai, Puei-Lene, et al. "Neurotrophic Properties of the Lion's Mane Medicinal Mushroom, *Hericium erinaceus* (Higher Basidiomycetes) from Malaysia." *International Journal of Medicinal Mushrooms* 15, no. 6 (2013): 539–54. https://doi.org/10.1615/intjmedmushr.v15.i6.30.

Lake, James. "S-Adenosyl-Methionine (SAMe) for Depressed Mood." *Psychology Today*, November 20, 2018.

Law, Kim Sooi, et al. "The Effects of Virgin Coconut Oil (VCO) as Supplementation on Quality of Life (QOL) among Breast Cancer Patients." *Lipids in Health and Disease* 13, no. 1 (2014). https://doi.org/10.1186/1476-511x-13-139.

Lekomtseva, Yevgeniya, Irina Zhukova, and Anna Wacker. "*Rhodiola rosea* in Subjects with Prolonged or Chronic Fatigue Symptoms: Results of an Open-Label Clinical Trial." *Complementary Medicine Research* 24, no. 1 (2017): 46–52. https://doi.org/10.1159/000457918.

Lenart, Kristof. "Magic Mushrooms and the Future of Mental Health Care." Canadian Nurse, July 2020.

Leung, M. C., et al. "Acupuncture Improves Cognitive Function: A Systematic

Review." *Neural Regeneration Research* 8, no. 18 (2013): 1673–84. doi:10.3969/j .issn.1673-5374.2013.18.005.

Levy, Jillian. "Aflatoxin Could Be in Your Peanut Butter & More." Dr. Axe, March 30, 2020.

Liaw, Fang-Yih, et al. "Exploring the Link between the Components of Metabolic Syndrome and the Risk of Depression." *BioMed Research International* 2015 (December 7, 2015): 1–8. https://doi.org/10.1155/2015/586251.

"Lighting Ergonomics—Light Flicker: OSH Answers." Canadian Centre for Occupational Health and Safety, May 13, 2021.

Lindberg, Sara. "Is Watching the News Bad for Mental Health?" Verywell Mind, May 18, 2020.

Link, Rachael. "Can This Fungi Fight Cancer?" Dr. Axe, September 20, 2019.

Lucatch, Aliya M., et al. "Cannabis and Mood Disorders." *Current Addiction Reports* 5, no. 3 (2018): 336–45. https://doi.org/10.1007/s40429-018-0214-y.

Madani, M., F. Tabatabaei, and Z. Tabatabaee. "The Relationship between Serum Vitamin D Level and Attention Deficit Hyperactivity Disorder." *Iranian Journal of Child Neurology* 9, no. 4 (2015): 48–53.

"Magnesium in Diet." MedlinePlus, May 4, 2021.

Main, Emily. "6 Facts About Farmed Shrimp That You Need to Know." *Good Housekeeping*, June 14, 2019.

Majumder, Irina, Jason M. White, and Rodney J. Irvine. "Antidepressant-Like Effects of Ecstasy in Subjects with a Predisposition to Depression." *Addictive Behaviors* 37, no. 10 (2012): 1189–92. https://doi.org/10.1016/j.addbeh.2012.05.022.

Malinowski, Peter. "Mindfulness Meditation: 10 Minutes a Day Improves Cognitive Function." Medical Xpress, September 19, 2018.

Mao, Jun J., et al. "*Rhodiola rosea* versus Sertraline for Major Depressive Disorder: A Randomized Placebo-Controlled Trial." *Phytomedicine* 22, no. 3 (2015): 394–99. https://doi.org/10.1016/j.phymed.2015.01.010.

Marie, Olive. "Study Finds Americans Don't Eat Adequate Fish, Missing Out on Health Benefits They Need." *Science Times*, November 14, 2020.

Marotta, Angela, et al. "Effects of Probiotics on Cognitive Reactivity, Mood, and Sleep Quality." *Frontiers in Psychiatry* 10 (2019). https://doi.org/10.3389/fpsyt.2019.00164.

Marshall, Amy Sarah. "The Detective Work of Autoimmune Disease." UVA Health, October 31, 2014.

Martínez Steele, Eurídice, et al. "Ultra-Processed Foods and Added Sugars in the US Diet: Evidence from a Nationally Representative Cross-Sectional Study." *BMJ Open* 6, no. 3 (2016). https://doi.org/10.1136/bmjopen-2015-009892.

Mayo Clinic Staff. "Meditation: A Simple, Fast Way to Reduce Stress." Mayo Clinic, April 22, 2020.

———. "St. John's Wort." Mayo Clinic, February 13, 2021.

McBride, Judy. "B_{12} Deficiency May Be More Widespread Than Thought: USDA ARS." US Department of Agriculture, August 2, 2000.

McCarthy, Claire. "Common Food Additives and Chemicals Harmful to Children." Harvard Health, July 24, 2018.

McIntyre, Roger S., et al. "Should Depressive Syndromes Be Reclassified as 'Metabolic Syndrome Type II'?" *Annals of Clinical Psychiatry* 19, no. 4 (2007): 257–64. https://doi.org/10.1080/10401230701653377.

"MDMA-Assisted Psychotherapy." Multidisciplinary Association for Psychedelic Studies, accessed May 14, 2021.

Meisner, Robert C., MD. "Ketamine for Major Depression: New Tool, New Questions." Harvard Medical School, May 22, 2019.

Melo, Helen M., Luís Eduardo Santos, and Sergio T. Ferreira. "Diet-Derived Fatty Acids, Brain Inflammation, and Mental Health." *Frontiers in Neuroscience* 13 (2019). https://doi.org/10.3389/fnins.2019.00265.

"Mind over Medicated." University of Vermont, July 6, 2019.

Mindworks Team. "How Meditation Changes the Brain." Mindworks, May 3, 2021.

Mischoulon, David. "Omega-3 Fatty Acids for Mood Disorders." Harvard Health, August 3, 2018.

"MTHFR Gene, Folic Acid, and Preventing Neural Tube Defects." Centers for Disease Control and Prevention, July 6, 2020.

Muthmainah and Ida Nurwati. "Acupuncture for Depression: The Mechanism Underlying Its Therapeutic Effect." *Medical Acupuncture* 28, no. 6 (2016): 301–7. https://doi.org/10.1089/acu.2016.1180.

Mutter, Rachel. "Here Are America's Most-Consumed Seafood Species." Intrafish, February 24, 2020.

Nawrat, Allie. "Psychedelics: A Game-Changer in Mental Health?" Pharmaceutical Technology, August 2020.

Nazario, Brunilda. "Ginseng for Your Immune System, Concentration, Heart, and Menopause." WebMD, September 26, 2020.

Newport, Cal. "Digital Addiction Getting You Down? Try an Analog Cure." *New York Times*, April 9, 2019.

"1 in 3 Adults Don't Get Enough Sleep." Centers for Disease Control and Prevention, February 16, 2016.

"One in Three Americans Has Metabolic Syndrome." CardioSmart, June 1, 2015. https://www.cardiosmart.org/news/2015/6/one-in-three-americans-has-metabolic-syndrome.

Opler, Lorne David. "Your Brain on Barbells: Could Strength Training Help Improve Your Mood?" *Washington Post*, September 2, 2020.

Patterson, E., et al. "Health Implications of High Dietary Omega-6 Polyunsaturated Fatty Acids." *Journal of Nutrition and Metabolism* 2012 (2012): 1–16. https://doi.org/10.1155/2012/539426.

"President's Council on Sports, Fitness & Nutrition." Homepage. President's Council on Sports, Fitness & Nutrition, accessed May 13, 2021.

People Staff. "Average U.S. Adult Will Spend Equivalent of 44 Years of Their Life Staring at Screens: Poll." *People*, June 3, 2020.

Phua, D. H., A. Zosel, and K. Heard. "Dietary Supplements and Herbal Medicine Toxicities—When to Anticipate Them and How to Manage Them." *International Journal of Emergency Medicine* 2, no. 2 (2009): 69–76. https://doi.org/10.1007/s12245-009-0105-z.

Pinto-Sanchez, Maria Ines, et al. "Probiotic *Bifidobacterium longum* NCC3001 Reduces Depression Scores and Alters Brain Activity: A Pilot Study in Patients With Irritable Bowel Syndrome." *Gastroenterology* 153, no. 2 (2017). https://doi .org/10.1053/j.gastro.2017.05.003.

Platero, Jose Luis, et al. "The Impact of Coconut Oil and Epigallocatechin Gallate on the Levels of IL-6, Anxiety and Disability in Multiple Sclerosis Patients." *Nutrients* 12, no. 2 (2020): 305. https://doi.org/10.3390/nu12020 0305.

Plourde, Mélanie, and Stephen C. Cunnane. "Extremely Limited Synthesis of Long Chain Polyunsaturates in Adults: Implications for Their Dietary Essentiality and Use as Supplements." *Applied Physiology, Nutrition, and Metabolism* 32, no. 4 (2007): 619–34. https://doi.org/10.1139/h07-034.

Preiato, Daniel. "Everything You Need to Know About 48-Hour Fasting." Healthline, May 23, 2019.

Preidt, Robert. "Many Common Meds Could Alter Your Microbiome." WebMD, October 23, 2019.

Price, Annie. "Butter Ingredient Contains Anti-Cancer Fat Shown to Induce Death of Colon Cancer Cells." Dr. Axe, March 27, 2020.

"Psychedelic Treatment with Psilocybin Relieves Major Depression, Study Shows." Johns Hopkins Medicine, November 4, 2020.

Rapaport, Mark Hyman, et al. "Massage Therapy for Psychiatric Disorders." *FOCUS* 16, no. 1 (2018): 24–31. https://doi.org/10.1176/appi.focus.20170043.

Rapoport, Stanley I. "Arachidonic Acid and the Brain." *Journal of Nutrition* 138, no. 12 (2008): 2515–20. https://doi.org/10.1093/jn/138.12.2515.

Reay, Jonathon L., David O. Kennedy, and Andrew B. Scholey. "Single Doses of Panax Ginseng (G115) Reduce Blood Glucose Levels and Improve Cognitive Performance during Sustained Mental Activity." *Journal of Psychopharmacology* 19, no. 4 (2005): 357–65. https://doi.org/10.1177/0269881105053286.

"Reducing Harmful Chemicals in Our Food." Environmental Defense Fund, accessed May 13, 2021.

Reinagel, Monica. "How Much Nutrition Do You Absorb from Food?" *Scientific American*, October 22, 2014.

Reis, Daniel J., Stephen S. Ilardi, and Stephanie E. Punt. "The Anxiolytic Effect of Probiotics: A Systematic Review and Meta-Analysis of the Clinical and Preclinical Literature." *PLoS ONE* 13, no. 6 (2018). https://doi.org/10.1371/journal.pone.0199041.

Reynolds, E. H. "Folic Acid, Ageing, Depression, and Dementia." *BMJ* 324, no. 7352 (2002): 1512–15. https://doi.org/10.1136/bmj.324.7352.1512.

Ríos-Hernández, Alejandra, et al. "The Mediterranean Diet and ADHD in Children and Adolescents." *Pediatrics* 139, no. 2 (2017). https://doi.org/10.1542/peds.2016-2027.

Roberts, Chris. "Proposed California Law Would Legalize Magic Mushrooms, MDMA, LSD, and Other Psychedelic Drugs." *Forbes*, February 19, 2021.

Roberts, Nicole F. "Americans Sit More Than Any Time in History and It's Literally Killing Us." *Forbes*, March 7, 2019.

Robinson, Jennifer. "Signs You're Low on Vitamin B_{12}." WebMD, April 25, 2020.

Robinson, Lawrence, and Melinda Smith. "Social Media and Mental Health." HelpGuide.org, April 19, 2021.

Robinson, Lawrence, Melinda Smith, and Jeanne Segal. "Smartphone Addiction." HelpGuide.org, April 19, 2021.

Rodriguez, Julia. "CDC Declares Sleep Disorders a Public Health Epidemic." Advanced Sleep Medicine Services, Inc., December 9, 2016.

Rodriguez, Tori. "Biofeedback Can Help Improve Symptoms of Mental Disorders." Psychiatry Advisor, December 17, 2018.

Ryu, Sun, et al. "*Hericium erinaceus* Extract Reduces Anxiety and Depressive Behaviors by Promoting Hippocampal Neurogenesis in the Adult Mouse Brain." *Journal of Medicinal Food* 21, no. 2 (2018): 174–80. https://doi.org/10.1089/jmf.2017.4006.

Säemann, Marcus D., et al. "Anti-Inflammatory Effects of Sodium Butyrate on Human Monocytes: Potent Inhibition of IL-12 and up-Regulation of IL-10 Production." *FASEB Journal* 14, no. 15 (2000): 2380–82. https://doi.org/10.1096/fj.00-0359fje.

Sammy, Melissa. "5 FDA-Approved Food Additives with Brain-Damaging Effects." MDLinx, 2020.

Sander, Libby. "The Case for Finally Cleaning Your Desk." *Harvard Business Review*, March 29, 2019.

"Schisandra." Memorial Sloan Kettering Cancer Center, June 29, 2020.

Schroeder, Michael. "What Eating Fermented Foods Does for Your Digestive Health." *U.S. News & World Report*, May 14, 2019.

"7 Reasons You Should Listen to Music When You Work Out." *HuffPost*, December 7, 2017.

Shiffer, Emily J. "Too Little Vitamin D Can Trigger Major and Minor Depression—Here's How to Add More Vitamin D to Your Diet." *Insider*, December 30, 2020.

Simon, E. B., et al. "Losing Neutrality: The Neural Basis of Impaired Emotional Control without Sleep." *Journal of Neuroscience* 35, no. 38 (2015): 13194–205. https://doi.org/10.1523/jneurosci.1314-15.2015.

———. "Overanxious and Underslept." *Nature Human Behaviour* 4, no. 1 (January 2020): 100–10.

Simopoulos, A. P. "The Importance of the Ratio of Omega-6/Omega-3 Essential Fatty Acids." *Biomedicine & Pharmacotherapy* 56, no. 8 (2002): 365–79. https://doi.org/10.1016/s0753-3322(02)00253-6.

Singer, Maya. "Could the Embrace of Psychedelics Lead to a Mental-Health Revolution?" *Vogue*, February 2021.

Singh, N., et al. "An Overview on Ashwagandha: A Rasayana (Rejuvenator) of Ayurveda." *African Journal of Traditional, Complementary and Alternative Medicines* 8, no. 5S (2011). https://doi.org/10.4314/ajtcam.v8i5s.9.

Sklar, Julia. "'Zoom Fatigue' Is Taxing the Brain. Here's Why That Happens." *National Geographic*, May 4, 2021.

"Sleep and Mood." Division of Sleep Medicine, Harvard Medical School, December 15, 2008.

"Social Media 'Likes' Impact Teens' Brains and Behavior." Association for Psychological Science, May 31, 2016.

Spencer, Sarah J., et al. "Food for Thought: How Nutrition Impacts Cognition and Emotion." *npj Science of Food* 1, no. 1 (2017). https://doi.org/10.1038/s41538-017-0008-y.

Spritzler, Franziska. "8 Signs and Symptoms of Vitamin D Deficiency." Healthline, July 23, 2018.

"The State of Sleep Health in America." Sleep Health, 2017.

Stoppler, Melissa Conrad. "Pain and Stress: Endorphins: Natural Pain and Stress Fighters." MedicineNet, June 13, 2018.

Sublette, M. Elizabeth. "Fatty Acid Levels in the Brain Are Found to Correlate with Serotonin Transport and Depression Severity." Brain & Behavior Research Foundation, February 14, 2020.

Sugg, Hayley. "3 Ways You're Sabotaging Your Probiotic Foods." *Cooking Light*, October 25, 2017.

Tiberian, Janet. "Americans Still Eating Too Many Low-Quality Carbs and Too Much Saturated Fat." MDVIP, December 14, 2019.

Tillisch, Kirsten, et al. "Consumption of Fermented Milk Product with Probiotic Modulates Brain Activity." *Gastroenterology* 144, no. 7 (2013). https://doi.org/10.1053/j.gastro.2013.02.043.

"Time for More Vitamin D." Harvard Medical School, July 27, 2020.

Tinsley, Grant. "6 Benefits of Reishi Mushroom (Plus Side Effects and Dosage)." Healthline, March 31, 2018.

Tiret, Holly. "Changing from Negative to Positive Thinking." Michigan State University, March 5, 2021.

Trasande, Leonardo. "Some Food Additives Raise Safety Concerns for Child Health; AAP Offers Guidance." American Academy of Pediatrics, May 11, 2021.

Troubat, Romain, et al. "Neuroinflammation and Depression: A Review." *European Journal of Neuroscience* 53, no. 1 (2020): 151–71. https://doi.org/10.1111/ejn.14720.

Tupper, Kenneth W., et al. "Psychedelic Medicine: A Re-Emerging Therapeutic Paradigm." *Canadian Medical Association Journal* 187, no. 14 (2015): 1054–59. https://doi.org/10.1503/cmaj.141124.

"2018 a Strong, Successful Year for U.S. Fishermen and Seafood Sector." National Oceanic and Atmospheric Administration. US Department of Commerce, 2018.

University of Kansas. "Want to Avoid the Holiday Blues? New Report Suggests Skipping the Sweet Treats." ScienceDaily, December 12, 2019.

University of Waterloo. "Just 10 Minutes of Meditation Helps Anxious People Have Better Focus." ScienceDaily, May 1, 2017.

Uwitonze, Anne Marie, and Mohammed S. Razzaque. "Role of Magnesium in Vitamin D Activation and Function." *Journal of the American Osteopathic Association* 118, no. 3 (2018): 181. https://doi.org/10.7556/jaoa.2018.037.

Van Dam, Romee, et al. "Lower Cognitive Function in Older Patients with Lower Muscle Strength and Muscle Mass." *Dementia and Geriatric Cognitive Disorders* 45, nos. 3–4 (2018): 243–50. https://doi.org/10.1159/000486711.

Vighi, G., et al. "Allergy and the Gastrointestinal System." *Clinical & Experimental Immunology* 153 (2008): 3–6. https://doi.org/10.1111/j.1365-2249.2008.03713.x.

Walker, Matthew P., and Els van der Helm. "Overnight Therapy? The Role of Sleep in Emotional Brain Processing." *Psychological Bulletin* 135, no. 5 (2009): 731–48. https://doi.org/10.1037/a0016570.

Wall, Rebecca, et al. "Bacterial Neuroactive Compounds Produced by Psychobiotics." *Advances in Experimental Medicine and Biology*, 2014, 221–39. https://doi.org/10.1007/978-1-4939-0897-4_10.

Wallace, Caroline J., and Roumen Milev. "The Effects of Probiotics on Depressive Symptoms in Humans: A Systematic Review." *Annals of General Psychiatry* 16, no. 1 (2017). https://doi.org/10.1186/s12991-017-0138-2.

Wallace, Kelly. "10 Signs You Might Be Addicted to Your Smartphone." CNN, January 9, 2015.

"Walnuts Are the Healthiest Nut, Say Scientists." BBC, March 27, 2011.

Wang, Huiying, et al. "Effect of Probiotics on Central Nervous System Functions in Animals and Humans: A Systematic Review." *Journal of Neurogastroenterology and Motility* 22, no. 4 (2016): 589–605. https://doi.org/10.5056/jnm16018.

Wani, Ab Latif, Sajad Ahmad Bhat, and Anjum Ara. "Omega-3 Fatty Acids and the Treatment of Depression: A Review of Scientific Evidence." *Integrative Medicine Research* 4, no. 3 (2015): 132–41. https://doi.org/10.1016/j.imr.2015.07.003.

Warner, Jennifer. "Low Vitamin B_6 Linked to Inflammation." WebMD, June 19, 2012.

Wei, Min, et al. "Fasting-Mimicking Diet and Markers/Risk Factors for Aging, Diabetes, Cancer, and Cardiovascular Disease." *Science Translational Medicine* 9, no. 377 (2017). https://doi.org/10.1126/scitranslmed.aai8700.

Weil, Andrew. "Siberian Ginseng." DrWeil.com, October 5, 2020.

Weng, Helen Y., et al. "Compassion Training Alters Altruism and Neural Responses to Suffering." *Psychological Science* 24, no. 7 (2013): 1171–80. https://doi.org/10.1177/0956797612469537.

"What America's Missing: A 2011 Report on the Nation's Nutrient Gap." Milk Processor Education Program, 2011.

Whitbread, Daisy. "Top 10 Foods Highest in Tryptophan." My Food Data, January 22, 2021.

"Why You Shouldn't Buy Supplements in the Grocery Store." Parsley Health, June 2, 2020.

Wilhelmi de Toledo, Françoise, et al. "Safety, Health Improvement and Well-Being during a 4- to 21-Day Fasting Period in an Observational Study Including 1422 Subjects." *PLoS ONE* 14, no. 1 (2019). https://doi.org/10.1371/journal.pone.0209353.

Winderl, Amy Marturana. "The 8 B Vitamins You Need and How to Get Them from Food." *Parsley Health Blog*, Parsley Health, December 16, 2019.

Wolf, Barney. "Quick Service's Push for Healthier Cooking Oils." *QSR*, 2017.

Wolfson, Philip E., et al. "MDMA-Assisted Psychotherapy for Treatment of Anxiety and Other Psychological Distress Related to Life-Threatening Illnesses: A Randomized Pilot Study." *Scientific Reports* 10, no. 1 (2020). https://doi.org/10.1038/s41598-020-75706-1.

Worland, Justin. "Digital Distraction: Cell Phones Distract Even When Not in Use." *Time*, December 4, 2014.

Wu, Suzanne. "Fasting Triggers Stem Cell Regeneration of Damaged, Old Immune System." *USC News*, University of Southern California, February 5, 2018.

Yang, Yan, et al. "Sedentary Behavior and Sleep Problems: A Systematic Review and Meta-Analysis." *International Journal of Behavioral Medicine* 24, no. 4 (2016): 481–92. https://doi.org/10.1007/s12529-016-9609-0.

Yao, Wei, et al. "Effects of Amycenone on Serum Levels of Tumor Necrosis Factor-α, Interleukin-10, and Depression-like Behavior in Mice after Lipopolysaccharide Administration." *Pharmacology Biochemistry and Behavior* 136 (2015): 7–12. https://doi.org/10.1016/j.pbb.2015.06.012.

Yeap, Swee Keong, et al. "Antistress and Antioxidant Effects of Virgin Coconut Oil in Vivo." *Experimental and Therapeutic Medicine* 9, no. 1 (2014): 39–42. https:// doi.org/10.3892/etm.2014.2045.

Yonezawa, Ken, et al. "Recent Trends in Mental Illness and Omega-3 Fatty Acids." *Journal of Neural Transmission* 127, no. 11 (2020): 1491–99. https://doi .org/10.1007/s00702-020-02212-z.

Zhang, Mingming, et al. "Effectiveness and Safety of Acupuncture for Insomnia." *Medicine* 98, no. 45 (2019). https://doi.org/10.1097/md.0000000000017842.

Zuckerman, Arthur. "Significant Yoga Statistics: 2020/2021 Benefits, Facts & Trends." CompareCamp.com, February 12, 2021.

———. "109 Technology Addiction Statistics: 2020/2021 Data, Facts & Insights." CompareCamp.com, February 12, 2021.

Index

A

acupuncture, 226, 230, 242, 251
adaptogenic herbs (adaptogens), 204
addictions
    alcohol and drug use and, 50, 58, 59
    mobile devices and social media use and,
        10, 55, 159, 160–61, 165–66, 171
    psychedelics for, 222, 223
    sugar and, 16
ADHD. *See* attention deficit hyperactivity
    disorder
adrenal glands
    diagnostic tests for, 74–76, 91
    function of, 73–74
advanced plan, 234
    description of, 246–52
    diagnostic tests before, 240, 245–48
    digital detox in, 242, 250
    eliminating inflammatory food groups in,
        240, 248
    meaningful movement in, 241, 249–50
    meditation and breathing in, 242, 250–51
    preparations before starting, 234–37
    progress assessment after completing, 252
    psychedelics in, 242, 251–52
    sleep planning in, 241–42, 250
    snapshot of, 240–42
    Supplement Starter Kit with, 240–41,
        248–49
aerobic exercise, 54–55, 105–6, 108–9, 238,
    241, 244
alcohol use. *See* substance misuse and abuse
Ambien, 12, 57, 103
American College of Sports Medicine, 114

antecedents, in ATMs approach, 17–18
antinuclear antibody (ANA) test, 81, 82, 91,
    237, 238, 246
antidepressants
    acupuncture and efficacy of, 230
    assessment for most effective class of, 91
    exercise compared with, 101–2
    psychedelics compared with, 214, 223,
        224
    vitamin B_{12} and folate levels and, 199
antithyroglobulin test, 73, 91, 240, 246
anti-thyroid peroxidase (TPO) test, 73, 81, 91,
    240, 246
anxiety
    acupuncture for, 230
    assessing your core actions' impact on, 48
    B vitamin levels and risk for, 53
    controlled movement schedule for, 110
    conventional medicine's approach to, 11
    coronavirus pandemic's impact on, 8
    craniosacral therapy and massage for, 229
    as a diagnosable medical condition, 8, 204
    diagnostic testing for causes of, 68, 69, 70
    exercise and movement for mood and, 107
    frequent diagnosis of, 7, 204
    genetic factors in, 77, 78
    high blood sugar levels and, 80
    intake screening for, 7
    Lyme disease and, 83
    normalization of, in American life, 9
    percentage of Americans experiencing, 8
    physical problems related to, 7, 8
    pop culture's portrayal of, 9
    prescription drugs for, 22, 24, 82, 225

anxiety (*cont.*)
    psychedelics for, 222–23, 225
    slow folate conversion and, 78
    supplements for, 189–90, 204–5, 240, 248
    technology and smartphones and, 56,
        167–68
    workout prescription for prevention and
        treatment of, 244
arachidonic acid (AA), 126
ashwagandha, 204, 205, 240, 248
ATMs (antecedents, triggers, and mediators),
    17–18
attention deficit hyperactivity disorder
    (ADHD)
    acupuncture for, 230
    assessing your core actions' impact on, 48
    conventional medicine's approach to, 11
    exercise and movement for, 99–100, 107
    frequent diagnosis of, 8
    high blood sugar levels and, 80
    percentage of Americans experiencing, 8
    technology and smartphones and, 169–71,
        173
autoimmune disorders, 89, 138. *See also*
    specific conditions
    elimination diet for, 248
    factors in, 81
    food sensitivity testing in, 150–51
    stage two immunity testing in, 82–84, 92
    thyroid function and, 72
autoimmune testing, 81–82, 91–92
ayahuasca, 212, 221

B

biofeedback, 226, 227–28, 242, 251
biotoxin illness test. *See* toxic mold illness test
blood sugar levels
    diagnostic testing for, 69, 70, 80–81, 91
    dietary sugar ingestion and, 51–52, 120
    inflammation from, 123–24
    stress's impact on, 105
    tests for, 80–81, 91
brain
    aerobic exercise and, 108
    alcohol use and, 59
    biofeedback therapy and, 227
    B vitamins and, 133–34, 135–36
    controlled movement and, 110
    dietary fats and oils and, 132–33
    elimination diet and, 147
    EPA and DHA levels and, 86, 126, 136
    fasting and, 143, 144, 145

food and diet and, 128–29, 131, 132
food sensitivities or intolerances and, 150
gut health and microbiome and, 88–89,
    136–37, 201
hormone disruptors in food and, 72
meditation and, 216, 217, 218, 246
mushrooms and, 141–42
plant-based paleo diet and, 128–29
probiotics and, 137, 201
sitting during technology use and, 110
sleep quality and processes in, 57, 102,
    103, 175
sugar consumption and, 10, 52, 80, 120,
    123–24
technology and smartphones and, 54, 55,
    165–66, 169, 172–73, 180
brain fog
    assessing your core actions' impact on, 48
    controlled movement schedule for, 110
    diagnostic testing for causes of, 68, 69, 70
    exercise and movement for mood and, 107
    frequent diagnosis of, 8
    genetic factors in, 77
    high blood sugar levels and, 80
    hormonal imbalances and, 77
    Lyme disease and, 83
    sleep quality and, 57
    technology and smartphones and, 169–70
breathing exercises
    in advanced plan, 250–51
    biofeedback and, 227
    in kickstarter plan, 239, 246
    meditation with, 217–18, 219, 221, 246
    tai chi with, 110
    yoga and, 3
breath test, for digestive health, 16, 23, 88, 89,
    90, 92, 247
burnout
    breathing exercises' impact on, 246
    controlled movement schedule for, 110
    conventional medicine's approach to, 11
    as a diagnosable medical condition, 8
    diagnostic testing for cause of, 67
    exercise and movement and, 107, 115
    frequent diagnosis of, 8
    normalization of, in American life, 9
    pop culture's portrayal of, 9
    stress's impact on, 105
    undiagnosed thyroid disorders and, 73
    workout prescription for, 244
B vitamins. *See also specific vitamins*
    deficiency or low levels of, 53, 85, 133

food sources of, 134, 135, 139
plant-based paleo diet with, 133–35
supplements for, 209

C

cardio exercise, 103, 105, 108–9, 218, 237, 244, 249–50
CDC, 78, 102, 103, 173
celiac disease, 134, 150, 201
Charon, Rita, 83
chronic fatigue, 78, 80, 83, 87, 109, 208, 226, 227, 230
coconut oil, 132, 133, 147, 154
Columbia Vagelos College of Physicians and Surgeons, 6, 11, 45–46
COMT gene variants
  supplements for, 79
  test for, 91, 240, 246
controlled movement, 106, 109–13, 238, 244. See also qigong; tai chi; yoga
core actions. See also diet and nutrition; exercise; sleep; substance misuse and abuse; technology and smartphone use
  as antecedents predating symptoms, 18
  changing for new baseline levels, 48–49
  definition of, 4
  interrelationship of, 60–61
  investigating impact on symptoms of, 42
  as mediators sustaining symptoms, 18
  patient interviews for impact of, 14, 22
  self-assessment of toxic impact of, 61–64
  shifting to achieve a State Change in, 5
cortisol
  adrenal production of, 73, 74
  five-point test for, 74, 91, 240, 246
  phosphatidylserine (PS) regulation of, 206
  sleep time and spikes in, 239, 241, 245
  stress response and, 74–75, 97, 105, 168, 174
COVID-19 (coronavirus) pandemic, 8, 101, 160, 162, 165, 178, 190
craniosacral therapy (CST), 226, 228–30, 242, 253
Crohn's disease, 25, 81, 84, 134, 201

D

daily behaviors. See core actions
dairy, in elimination diet, 153, 155
Davidson, Richard, 173
depression
  acupuncture for, 230
  assessing your core actions' impact on, 48

B vitamin levels and risk for, 53
  conventional medicine's approach to, 11
  coronavirus pandemic's impact on, 8
  craniosacral therapy and massage for, 229
  diagnostic testing for causes of, 67, 68, 69, 70
  energy work for, 227
  exercise and movement for, 54–55, 107
  frequent diagnosis of, 8
  genetic factors in, 77, 78
  high blood sugar levels and, 80
  hormonal imbalances and, 77
  intake screening for, 7
  Lyme disease and, 83
  meditation for, 216–17
  percentage of Americans experiencing, 8
  physical problems related to, 7, 8
  pop culture's portrayal of, 9
  psychedelics for, 222–23, 224
  slow folate conversion and, 78
  sugar in diet and, 52
  technology and smartphones and, 167–68
DHA (docosahexaenoic acid), 86, 87, 126, 198, 200, 238, 244
diabetes, 10, 47, 69, 80
diagnostic tests, 65–93. See also specific tests
  adrenals and, 73–76, 91
  in advanced plan, 240, 245–48
  autoimmune testing and, 81–82, 91–92
  blood sugar levels and, 80–81, 91
  cheat sheet for requests for, 71, 90–92
  digestive health testing in, 88–90, 92
  examples of using, 23, 67–68
  genetic testing and, 77–79, 91
  in kickstarter plan, 237, 238
  lack of a primary care doctor and omission of, 25
  nutrient deficiency testing and, 84–87, 92
  ordering, based on Parsley Symptom Index, 42
  Parsley Symptom Index compared with, 30
  primary doctors and, 66–67, 69–70
  psychiatrists and, 70
  sex hormones and, 76–77, 91
  stage two immunity testing in, 82–84, 92
  thyroid conditions and, 67–68, 71–73, 91
diet and nutrition, 117–57
  balancing blood sugar in, 123, 124–25
  benefits of, 127
  blood sugar impact of, 51–52, 120
  elimination diet and, 147–57

diet and nutrition (*cont.*)
    emotional health related to, 122–23
    energy and flow and, 50–53, 123–27
    fasting and, 143–47
    food allergies, intolerances, and
        sensitivities and, 52–53, 123
    gut-healing protocol in, 23, 24
    heart disease and, 120
    impact of processed foods in, 51, 53,
        120–22
    industrial food chemicals in, 121, 125,
        126–27, 128
    interrelationship of other core actions
        with, 60–61
    ketogenic diet and, 129–30
    mood and, 123
    plant-based paleo diet in, 128–43
    right types of fat in, 123, 125–26
    salt in, 127–28
    self-assessment of toxic impact of, 61–64
    State Change and, 5
    sugar and. *See* sugar in diet
    three things mattering most in, 123
    thyroid function and chemicals in, 72
digestive health testing, 88–90, 92
digital detox
    in advanced plan, 242, 250
    description of, 183–85
    in kickstarter plan, 239, 245–46
digital devices. *See* technology and
    smartphone use
DNA tests, 78
drug use. *See* substance misuse and abuse

E

eleuthero, 208–9
elimination diet, 147–57
    in advanced plan, 240, 248
    benefits of, 147
    food intolerances and, 149–50
    foods eaten for thirty days in, 153–54
    foods eliminated for thirty days in, 151–52
    food sensitivity versus food allergy and,
        148–49
    in kickstarter plan, 237, 238, 243
    meal suggestions on, 155–57
    misconceptions about, 148
    reintroducing foods in, 154–55
    withdrawal symptoms in, 154
emotional health
    body as fundamental driver of, 14
    coronavirus pandemic's impact on, 8

    Parsley Health's interest in a patient's
        experience of, 7–8
    physical health related to, 9–10
    State Change in. *See* State Change
emotional issues
    breathing exercises' impact on, 246
    normalization of, in American life, 8–9
    percentage of Americans experiencing, 8
emotions, sleep and processing of, 97–98, 99,
    100, 108–9
endorphins, and exercise, 54, 99, 105, 108
energy, low levels of. *See* fatigue and tiredness
energy and flow, 49–64
    assessing your core actions' impact on, 48
    exercise for, 53–55
    five core actions impacting, 49–50
    food for, 50–53, 123–27
    self-assessment of core actions blocking,
        61–64
    sleep for, 56–58
    substance misuse and abuse and, 58–60
    supplements for, 208–9
    technology and smartphone use and,
        55–56
    using tools for gradual change in, 60–61
energy healing, 228
energy work, 225–30
    acupuncture and, 230
    biofeedback and, 227–28
    craniosacral therapy and massage and,
        228–30
    energy meridians in, 225–26
    reiki and, 228
EPA (eicosapentaenoic acid), 86, 87, 126, 198,
    200, 238, 244
Epstein-Barr virus (EBV) test, 82, 83, 92,
    240, 247
erythrocyte sedimentation rate (ESR) test, 81,
    92, 237, 238, 246
estrogen test, 69, 71, 76, 77, 91, 240, 246
exercise, 97–115
    ADHD symptoms and, 99–100
    advanced plan with, 241, 249–50
    aerobic, 54–55, 105–6, 108–9, 238, 241, 244
    antidepressants compared with, 101–2
    benefits of, 54, 99, 101–6
    cardio workouts in, 103, 105, 108–9, 218,
        237, 244, 249–50
    controlled movement in, 106, 109–13,
        238, 244
    depression and, 54–55, 107
    energy and flow and, 53–55

interrelationship of other core actions with, 60–61
kickstarter plan with, 238–39, 244–45
mental health and, 54, 99–101
mindset shifts needed for, 107–8
mood and, 54–55, 101
necessity of, 54, 104–6
prescription for, 106–15
processing of emotions and, 97–98, 99, 100, 108–9
self-assessment of impact of lack of, 61–64
sleep and, 102–4
strength-building workouts in, 106, 108, 113–15, 237, 239, 241, 244–45, 249
extra-virgin olive oil (EVOO), 132–33

F

fasting, 143–47
fasting sprints or keto sprints, 145, 147
intermittent, 143
Morning Glory Coffee and, 146
prolonged, 144–46
fasting glucose test, 80–81, 91, 237, 238
fasting insulin test, 80–81, 91, 237, 238
fasting sprints, 145
fatigue and tiredness
acupuncture for, 230
chronic, 78, 80, 83, 87, 109, 208, 226, 227, 230
conventional medicine's approach to, 11
cortisol levels and, 75
craniosacral therapy and massage for, 229
diagnostic testing for causes of, 67, 68, 69, 70
energy work for, 227
frequent diagnosis of, 7
high blood sugar levels and, 80
hormonal imbalances and, 77
intake screening for, 7
Lyme disease and, 83
percentage of Americans experiencing, 8
physical problems related to, 7, 8
slow folate conversion and, 78
workout prescription for prevention of, 244
fats, dietary, 132, 133, 147
elimination diet with, 154
plant-based paleo diet with, 132–33, 135–36
right kind for diet, 123, 125–26
ferritin
anemia and iron deficiency and, 85, 87
deficiency test for, 85, 92, 237, 238

5-hydroxytryptophan (5-HTP), 207, 241, 249
five-point cortisol test, 74, 91, 240, 246
FLC (Feel Like Crap) syndrome, 52
folate, deficiency test for, 92, 237, 238
food. *See* diet and nutrition
food allergy, versus food sensitivity, 148–49
food intolerances, 52–53, 123, 149–50, 151
food sensitivities, 123
food allergy versus, 148–49
elimination diet and, 150–51
gluten and, 52–53, 148, 150, 155, 243
impact of, 52–53
testing for, 150–51
free T3 (triiodothyronine) test, 91, 237, 238
free T4 (thyroxine) test, 91, 237, 238

G

GABA (gamma-aminobutyric acid), 190, 205–6, 241, 249
genetic testing, 77–79, 91. *See also* COMT gene variants; MTHFR gene variants
ghee, 132, 133
ginseng, 204, 208–9
glucose, fasting test for, 80–81, 91, 237, 238
gluten
elimination diet and, 23, 152, 154–55, 238, 242, 243, 248
sensitivity to, 52–53, 148, 150, 155, 243
gluten-free diet and foods, 15, 235, 248
Goenka, Satya Narayan, 96–97, 98
Graves's disease, 73
gut health. *See also* microbiome
testing for, 88–90, 92

H

Hashimoto's thyroiditis, 67–68, 73, 81–82
health. *See also* emotional health
Parsley Symptom Index for evaluating, 29
story of your life and story of, 17, 22, 66
taking responsibility for, 16–17
health biography, 15–16, 18–20, 42
hemoglobin A1C (HgBA1C) test, 80, 91, 237, 238
high-sensitivity C-reactive protein (hsCRP) test, 81, 92, 237, 238, 246
hormone testing, 71. *See also specific tests*
hydrogen/methane breath test, 16, 23, 88, 89, 90, 92, 247
Hyman, Dr. Mark, 52
hypothalamus-pituitary-adrenal (HPA) axis, 76
hypothyroidism, 68, 71, 72, 73, 84

I

insomnia, 8, 48, 227
Institute for Functional Medicine, 247
insulin, fasting test for, 80–81, 91, 237, 238
insulin resistance, 80
intermittent fasting, 143
iodine
    deficiency test for, 92, 240, 246
    thyroid function and, 72, 85
irritable bowel syndrome (IBS), 21–22,
        23–24, 84, 90, 230

K

ketamine, 58, 212, 221–22, 224
ketogenic diet, 129–30
keto sprints, 130, 145, 147
kickstarter plan, 233
    benefits of, 236
    breathing exercises in, 239, 250–51
    description of, 237–39, 242–45
    diagnostic tests before, 237, 238
    digital detox in, 239, 245–46
    eliminating inflammatory food groups in,
        237, 238, 243
    meaningful movement in, 238–39,
        244–45
    meditation in, 239, 245–46
    preparations before starting, 234–37
    progress assessment after completing, 252
    sleep planning in, 239, 245
    snapshot of, 238–39
    Supplement Starter Kit with, 238,
        243–44
    when to use, 234, 235

L

Longo, Dr. Valter, 144
LSD, 212, 221–22
L-theanine, 190, 205–6, 241, 249
Lyme disease test, 82, 83, 92, 240, 247

M

magnesium
    deficiency test for, 92, 240, 246
    plant-based paleo diet with, 140–41
    supplements containing, 205, 241, 249
magnesium glycinate, 205, 241, 249
magnesium threonate, 205, 241, 249
marijuana (pot), 58, 59, 211. See also
        substance misuse and abuse
massage, 226, 228–30, 242, 253

mediators, in ATMs approach, 17–18
meditation, 215–21
    in advanced plan, 242, 250–51
    brain changes using, 216, 217, 218, 246
    breathing practice with, 217–18, 219, 221,
        239, 246, 250–51
    depression treatment using, 216–17
    finding the right approach to, 217–19
    forms of, 220
    in kickstarter plan, 239, 245–46
    releasing emotions using, 99
    resource guide to, 219–20
    Vipassana and, 96–99
melatonin, 56, 137, 174, 175, 245
memory loss, and technology use, 171–73
mental health
    assessing your core actions' impact on, 48
    conventional medicine's approach to, 11
    exercise and, 54, 99, 101
    food sensitivities and, 52–53
    Parsley Health's interest in a patient's
        experience of, 7–8
    relationships and, 49–50
mental health disorders
    B vitamin levels and, 133, 134
    diagnostic testing for conditions in, 70
    energy work for, 227
    pop culture's portrayal of, 9
    prevalence of Americans experiencing, 8
    psychedelics for, 222, 223, 224–25
    sleep quality and, 57
    smartphone and technology use and,
        55–56, 159, 162–63, 167–69
metabolic syndrome Type II, 52
methylated B_{12} supplement, 79, 188, 198,
        199–200, 207, 238, 244
methylated B vitamins, 79, 87, 198–99, 209
methylated folate supplement, 79, 188,
        199–200, 207, 238, 244
microbiome
    functions of, 88–89
    high blood sugar levels and, 80
    plant-based paleo diet and, 136–38
micronutrients. See nutrients
mind-body connection, 12
MDMA (midomafetamine), 212, 221–22, 223,
        225
mold toxic illness, test for, 82, 83, 84, 92, 240,
        247
mood
    assessing your core actions' impact on, 48
    controlled movement schedule for, 110

exercise and, 54–55, 101, 109
food sensitivities and, 52–53
hormonal imbalances and, 77
omega-3 fat deficiency and, 53
sleep quality and, 57–58
smartphone and technology use and, 55–56
substance misuse and abuse and, 58, 60
sugar intake and, 51–52, 54
supplements targeting issues in, 203–7
undiagnosed thyroid disorders and, 73
mood disorders
craniosacral therapy and massage for, 229
energy work for, 227
genetic factors in, 78
psychedelics for, 222, 223, 224, 225
reiki for, 228
ultrarefined foods in, 53
Morning Glory Coffee, 146
movement. *See also* exercise
advanced plan with, 241, 249–50
kickstarter plan with, 238–39, 244–45
MTHFR gene variants
B vitamins and, 78–79, 134, 188, 199
mood and, 78, 199
supplements for, 79, 87, 188, 199–200
test for, 79, 87, 91, 246
Multidisciplinary Association for Psychedelic Studies (MAPS), 222
mushrooms, in plant-based paleo diet, 141–42
mushrooms, magic (psilocybin), 58, 212–14, 221, 222–23

N
neurosurgery, 45–46
Newport, Cal, 181
nutrient deficiencies. *See also specific deficiencies*
testing for, 84–87, 92
nutrients. *See also specific nutrients*
processed foods and lack of, 53
thyroid function and, 72
nutrition. *See* diet and nutrition

O
oils, dietary
elimination diet with, 154
plant-based paleo diet with, 132–33
olive oil, 132–33, 147, 154
omega-3 fats, 53, 76, 84, 125–26
plant-based paleo diet with, 135–36
supplements with, 198, 200

omega-3 index, 86, 92, 240, 246
omega-3 supplements, 198, 200, 238, 244
Oz, Dr. Mehmet, 118–19, 122

P
paleo diet. *See* plant-based paleo diet
Panax ginseng, 204, 208–9
Parsley Health
blog by, 237
body as fundamental driver of emotional health and, 14
breathing practice at, 219
diagnostic tests at, 67, 71, 74, 78, 79, 81, 82, 83, 88, 247
digital device use and, 163–64
elimination diet used by, 139, 147
food sensitivity testing at, 150
learning about a patient's mental and emotional health at, 7–8
nutrition deficiencies seen at, 85, 199
online links for, 247
plant-based paleo diet used by, 128
probiotic used by, 202
questionnaire on toxic effects of core actions used by, 61–62
State Change and outcomes at, 233
supplements used at, 191, 202, 204
Parsley Symptom Index (PSI), 28–43
baseline and, 48
body systems and possible symptoms covered in, 31
description of, 28
diagnostic testing compared with, 30
finding your symptom score on, 39
how to complete, 31
identifying impact of core actions using, 61–64
kickstarter plan and score on, 234
next steps for symptoms identified on, 41–43
questions in, 32–39
rating symptoms in, 31
recognizing patterns in, 29–30
self-assessment after completing plans using, 252
understanding your symptom score on, 40–41
ways of using results from, 28–30
peyote, 212, 221
phone use. *See* technology and smartphone use
phosphatidylserine (PS), 206

plans. *See* advanced plan; kickstarter plan

plant-based paleo diet, 128–43
  benefits of, 129
  brain-friendly fats in, 132–33
  brain-friendly oils in, 135–36
  brain impact of, 128–29
  B vitamins in, 133–35
  commercial "paleo" products and, 143
  core actions in, 128
  definition and description of, 130–31
  eleven approaches to, 131–43
  keto sprints in, 130
  leafy green vegetables in, 131–32
  magnesium in, 140–41
  microbiome and, 136–38
  mushrooms in, 141–42
  nuts and seeds for metabolism in, 139–40
  resetting sugar preference in, 138–39
  whole grains in, 142

post-EBV inflammatory syndrome, 83

post-traumatic stress disorder (PTSD), 222, 223

post-treatment Lyme disease syndrome
  (PTLDS), 83

pre-addiction phase, 59

prescription drugs
  acupuncture and efficacy of, 230
  antecedents predating symptoms with, 18
  average number per American, 10
  B vitamins and folates and, 199
  conventional medicine's use of, 13
  COVID-19 pandemic and use of, 101
  exercise compared with, 101, 103, 107
  genetics for personalizing, 78
  gut microbes affected by, 137, 202
  healthcare structure and, 48
  patients' experiences lowering dosage of,
    23–24, 90
  percentage of Americans taking, 13
  psychedelics compared with, 214, 223,
    224, 231
  sleeping disorders and, 57, 103, 104
  supplements and, 187, 188, 192, 206, 209
  triggers provoking symptoms and, 18

primary care doctors
  cheat sheet for requests for, 71, 90–92
  conventional critical care approach versus
    prevention and, 47–48
  diagnostic testing by, 66–67, 69–70, 80
  learning about a patient's mental and
    emotional health by, 7–8
  stereotypes about, 46
  undetected health issues from lack of, 25

probiotics
  brain and, 137, 201
  supplements with, 199, 201–3

processed and refined foods
  elimination diet and, 151, 155
  impact of, 51, 120–21
  plant-based paleo diet and, 128
  vitamins, nutrients, and other elements
    missing in, 53, 121–22

progesterone test, 71, 76, 77, 91, 240, 246

prolonged fasting, 144–46

PSI. *See* Parsley Symptom Index

psilocybin (magic mushrooms), 58, 212–14,
  221, 222–23

psychedelic medicines, 58, 221–25
  in advanced plan, 242, 251–52
  examples of use of, 211–14, 225
  integration therapy used with, 224–25
  ketamine and, 224
  magic mushrooms and, 222–23
  MDMA and, 223
  sources of, 221–22

psychiatric drugs, 12, 101, 102, 209, 230

psychiatrists
  clinical psychedelic treatment and, 251
  diagnostic testing used by, 70
  functional, with online practices, 248
  genetics for personalizing prescriptions
    from, 78
  separation of physical health and mental
    health by, 11–12, 21, 25, 26, 70

psychobiotics, 137, 202

pyridoxal 5-phosphate (P5P), 209

pyridoxine (vitamin B$_6$), 134–35, 209

Q

qigong, 106, 109–11, 112, 113, 238, 244–45

R

reiki, 226, 228, 242, 251

Rhodiola rosea, 208, 241, 249, 294

Robbins, Tony, 233

S

St. John's wort, 206–7, 241, 249

salt, dietary, 127–28

SAMe (S-adenosylmethionine), 207, 241, 249

schisandra, 204, 205, 240, 248

selenium
  deficiency test for, 92, 240, 246
  thyroid function and, 72, 85

serotonin
   depression or anxiety and lack of, 82
   foods and vitamins necessary for, 53, 78,
      135, 140, 207
   microbiome's control of, 52, 88, 124, 137,
      201
   neuroinflammation's blocking of, 126, 200
   psychedelics and, 221, 223
sex hormones. *See also specific hormones*
   diagnostic testing for, 76–77, 91
sleep
   advanced plan and, 241–42, 250
   brain processing during, 57
   energy and flow and, 56–58
   exercise as an aid to, 102–4
   interrelationship of other core actions
      with, 60–61
   kickstarter plan and, 239, 245
sleep disorders
   acupuncture for, 230
   craniosacral therapy and massage for, 229
   example of, 103–4
   health impact of, 57–58
   hormonal imbalances and, 77
   impact of, 103
   intake screening for, 7
   melatonin disruption from technology use
      and, 56, 174
   percentage of Americans experiencing, 8
   physical problems related to, 7
   prescription drugs and, 57, 103, 104
   self-assessment of toxic impact of, 61–64
   stress's impact on, 105
   supplements for, 205, 241, 249
   technology and smartphones and, 173–75,
      177–78
small intestine bacterial overgrowth (SIBO),
   16, 89–90
smartphone use. *See* technology and
   smartphone use
social media. *See also* technology and
   smartphone use
   addictive qualities of, 55
   digital detox from, 183–85
   mental health impact of, 55–56, 167–68,
      169
   setting a daily limit on, 176–77
sodium, dietary, 127–28
Starter Kit for supplements, 198–203
State Change
   core actions and, 5
   definition of, 4

implementing across daily life, 253–54
   reevaluating the rest of your life after, 6
stool test, for digestive health, 88, 90, 92,
   240, 247
strength building, 106, 108, 113–15, 237, 239,
   241, 244–45, 249
stress
   breathing exercises' impact on, 219, 246
   coronavirus pandemic's impact on, 8
   cortisol response to, 74–75, 97, 105, 168, 174
   meditation for, 217
   pre-addiction phase in dealing with, 59
   technology and smartphones and, 56,
      167–69
substance misuse and abuse
   energy and flow and, 58–60
   interrelationship of other core actions
      with, 60–61
   line between use, abuse, and addiction in,
      50, 58
   occasional healthy use versus, 58–59
   pre-addiction phase in, 59
   self-assessment of toxic impact of, 61–64
sugar in diet
   addictive aspect of, 16
   blood sugar impact of, 51–52, 120
   B vitamin depletion and, 199
   elimination diet and, 139, 147, 148, 150,
      151–52, 155, 238, 240, 243, 248
   fruits and, 153
   impact of, 123–24, 243
   microbiome health and, 202
   mood disorders and, 51–52, 54
   plant-based paleo diet and, 128, 129, 131,
      138–39, 143
   probiotic foods with, 202
   processed foods with, 120–21, 122, 151–52
   resetting taste preference for, 138–39
   self-assessment of amount of, 235
   thyroid conditions related to, 72
   typical food amounts of, 124–25
   ultrarefined foods with, 51
   unhealthy gut and, 89
supplements, 187–209. *See also specific
      supplements*
   for anxiety, 189–90, 204–5, 240, 248
   for calm, 203, 204–6
   example of use of, 189–90
   for energy and focus, 203, 208–9
   gut-healing diet with, 23, 24
   hypothalamus-pituitary-adrenal axis
      regulation and, 76

supplements (*cont.*)
  for mood burst, 203, 206–7
  mood issues and, 203–7
  MTHFR variant and, 79, 87, 188, 199–200
  for sleep problems, 205, 241, 249
  things to know about, 190–98
Supplement Starter Kit
  advanced plan and, 240–41, 248–49
  kickstarter plan and, 238, 243–44
  snapshot of, 198–203
symptom index. *See* Parsley Symptom Index

T

tai chi, 105, 106, 109, 110–11, 112, 113, 238,
      244
technology and smartphone use, 159–85
  addictive qualities of, 10, 55, 159, 160–61,
      165–66, 171
  ADHD and, 169–71, 173
  in advanced plan, 242, 250
  anxiety and depression with, 167–69
  brain changes from, 56, 173, 180
  brain fog and, 169–70
  designating a screen-free day and, 182–83
  digital detox in, 183–85, 239, 250, 245–46
  energy and flow and, 55–56
  examples of, 159–62, 170–71
  high-impact ways to change your
      relationship with, 180–85
  interrelationship of other core actions
      with, 60–61
  in kickstarter plan, 239, 245–46
  melatonin disruption from, 56, 174
  memory loss and, 171–73
  mental health impact of, 55–56, 159,
      162–63, 167–69
  planning analog activities versus, 180–81
  putting your phone away and, 180
  rebooting your relationship with, 176–80
  screen time use in, 164–65
  self-assessment of toxic impact of, 61–64
  setting a daily limit on, 176–77
  sleep problems and, 173–75, 177–78
  stress levels and, 56
  using audio calls only, 178–79

testosterone test, 69, 71, 76, 77, 91, 240, 246
three-day stool test, 88, 90, 92, 240, 247
thyroid conditions, 68, 71–73, 91
thyroid-stimulating hormone (TSH), 72–73,
      91, 237, 238
tiredness. *See* fatigue and tiredness
toxic mold illness test, 82, 83, 84, 92, 240,
      247
transcendental meditation, 221
triggers, in ATMs approach, 17–18

V

Vipassana, 96–99, 220
vitamin B_5, 134–35
vitamin B_6, 134–35, 209
vitamin B_{12} deficiency test, 92, 237, 238
vitamin D_3
  deficiency test for, 92, 237, 238
  supplements for, 198, 200–201
vitamins. *See specific vitamins*

W

warrior variant of COMT gene, 79
World Health Organization, 8
worrier variant of COMT gene, 79

Y

yoga, 54, 105
  benefits of, 5, 60, 112, 113
  exercise prescription using, 106, 107,
      109–11, 244
  increasing frequency or duration of,
      249–50
  kickstarter plan with, 238
  meditation and, 218, 221
  patient's experience with, 111–12
  State Change with, 3–5, 117

Z

zinc
  deficiency test for, 92, 240, 246
  thyroid function and, 72, 85
Zoloft, 12, 24, 54–55, 82, 207, 225
zolpidem (Ambien), 12, 57, 103

About the Author

Dr. Robin Berzin is the founder and CEO of Parsley Health, America's leading holistic medical practice designed to help people overcome chronic conditions. She founded Parsley to address the rising tide of chronic disease in America through personalized holistic medicine that puts food, lifestyle, and proactive diagnostic testing on the prescription pad next to medications. Since founding Parsley in 2016, Dr. Berzin has seen 80 percent of patients improve or resolve their chronic conditions within their first year of care, demonstrating the life-changing value of making modern holistic medicine accessible to everyone, everywhere. Parsley is available online nationwide.

Dr. Berzin attended medical school at Columbia University and trained in internal medicine at Mount Sinai Hospital in New York City. She has been recognized by the World Economic Forum as a Technology Pioneer and named to *Inc.* magazine's Female Founders 100 list, and Parsley Health was named to *Fast Company's* Most Innovative Companies list.

Parsley Health

Parsley Health is the nation's leading holistic medical practice, designed to help women overcome chronic conditions. Eighty percent of Parsley Health patients find relief within their first year of care—improving or resolving conditions like IBS, infertility, anxiety, and autoimmune disorders.

At Parsley, patients see the whole picture of their health, identify and address the root drivers of illness, and experience accessible and supportive care from providers who listen. As a result, patients feel better and have a true partner in improving and managing their health. Parsley Health is available online nation-wide and is the first one-stop shop for women's chronic care and holistic health.

Learn more about Parsley Health and get exclusive offers at parsleyhealth.com/statechange.